In Search of Manna

In Search of Manna

"Your Guide to Glyconutrients and Meridians"

M. Schlachter, MD
T. Aristotle, D.C., L.Ac.

Sano Press
1930 Village Center Circle
Suite 3-177
Las Vegas, Nevada 89134

Library of Congress Number: 2003094616 (cataloging in progress)

ISBN: 0-9743151-0-9

Printed in the United States of America

Our fathers did eat manna in the desert;
as it is written,
He gave them
bread from heaven to eat.

John 6:31

TABLE OF CONTENTS

PART I: Introduction 1

Read This First – How to Use this Book..3
A Personal Message from Dr. Schlachter 4
A Personal Message from Dr. Aristotle..5
Emergency and Maintenance Menu Definitions...........................6
Healing Reactions..7
Tips to Handle Healing Reactions..8
What to do about Specific Diseases..9
Glyco-Meridian Therapy™ the Hospital Environment 10
Rules for Meridian Point Stimulation 12

PART II: Conditions...13

Abdominal Pain..14
Abscess, Skin..15
Acne..16
Actinic Keratosis 17
ADD w/Hyperactivity...18
Addiction 19
Adrenal Exhaustion...20
Adrenal Insufficiency (Addison's Disease).................................21
Adult Respiratory Distress Syndrome (ARDS)............................22
AIDS 23
Alcohol Abuse 24
Allergic Rhinitis...25
Allergy...26
Alopecia...27
ALS (Amyotrophic Lateral Sclerosis).......................................28
Alzheimer's (Dementia) 29
Amalgam Toxicity 30
Amenorrhea 31
Amyotrophic Lateral Sclerosis (ALS)..32
Anemia 33
Anemia, Sickle Cell...34
Aneurysm (Aortic)...35
Angina Pectoris 36
Angioneurotic Edema 37
Ankylosing Spondylitis (AS) 38
Anorexia...39
Anorexia Nervosa 40
Antihistamine..41
Anxiety State...42
Aphthous Ulcer (Canker Sore) 43
Arrhythmia 44
Arterial Insufficiency 45

Arthralgia...46
Arthritis 47
AS (Ankylosing Spondylitis) 48
ASHD/CAD (Atherosclerotic Heart Disease) 49
Asthma w/o Status Asthmaticus 50
Athlete's Foot 51
Atrial Fibrillation.......................................52
Atrial Flutter 53
Attention Deficit Disorder (ADD) 54
Autism 55
Back Pain w/ Radiation................................56
Bacteremia (Not Septicemia) 57
Bacterial Infection 58
Bed Sores..59
Bell's Palsy...60
Bipolar Affective Disorder 61
Bladder Problems 62
Bloating / Flatulence / Gas...........................63
Blocked Tear Duct Lacrimal Duct Obstruction 64
Blood Pressure (Elevated w/o Hypertension) 65
Blood Sugar (Low) 66
Bowel Detoxification 67
Breast Cyst 68
Breast Implants (Leaking)..............................69
Bronchiectasis 70
Bronchitis, Chronic 71
Bruise Easily..72
Burns 73
Bursitis..74
Cancer 75
Candidiasis 76
Candidiasis (Oral).......................................77
Canker Sores 78
Cardiomyopathy..79
Cellulitis Abscess 80
Cerebral Aneurysm (Nonruptured) 81
Cerebral Arteriosclerosis...............................82
Cerebral Hemorrhage (Intracranial)...................83
Cerebrovascular Disease 84
Cervical Dysplasia......................................85
Cervicitis..86
Chest Wall Pain (Costochondritis) 87
Chickenpox...88
Chlamydia...89
Cholecystitis (Acute) 90
Cholecystitis (Chronic)................................91
Chronic Fatigue Syndrome 92
Chronic Ischemic Heart Disease 93
Chronic Liver Disease..................................94
Chronic Skin Ulcer Venous Stasis 95

Cirrhosis, Alcoholic Liver 96
Cirrhosis, Nonalcoholic Liver 97
Claudication/Peripheral Vascular Disease 98
Clostridium Difficile...99
Cold Sores...100
Cold/Flu 101
Colitis 102
Colon Infection 103
Coma 104
Common Cold 105
Concussion 106
Congenital Heart Defect..107
Congestive Heart Failure (CHF).....................................108
Conjunctivitis..109
Connective Tissue Disease 110
Constipation 111
Contact Dermatitis 112
COPD..113
Cor Pulmonale 114
Costochondritis 115
Cough 116
Coumadin Therapy (Long Term).....................................117
Cramps (Menstrual)..118
Cravings (Sweets/Alcohol) 119
Crohn's Disease 120
Croup 121
Cushing's Syndrome..122
CVA / Stroke..123
Cystitis (Acute UTI)...124
Cystitis (Chronic)..125
Cysts- Breasts...126
Cytomegalovirus..127
Dandruff 128
Decubitus Ulcer 129
Deep Vein Thrombosis (DVT) 130
Degenerative Disc Disease 131
Degenerative Joint Disease (DJD) 132
Depression 133
Dermatitis, Atopic Eczema..134
Detoxification (Systemic)...135
Diabetes...136
Diabetic Sores 137
Diarrhea 138
Diverticulitis w/o Hemorrhage.......................................139
Dizziness (Vertigo) 140
DJD (Degenerative Joint Disease) 141
Drug Addiction...142
Duodenal Ulcer 143
DVT (Deep Vein Thrombosis) 144
Dyslexia 145

Dyspepsia 146
Dyspnea.. 147
Dysuria... 148
Earache 149
Elevated Blood Pressure w/o Hypertension................... 150
Emphysema 151
Endocarditis (Acute/Subacute Bacterial) 152
Endocervicitis... 153
Endometriosis 154
Enteritis (Bacterial) 155
Enterocolitis, Ulcerative, Chronic.............................. 156
Epstein-Barr Virus 157
Esophageal Spasm 158
Esophagitis 159
Eustachian Tube Infection....................................... 160
Excessive Sweating (Hyperhidrosis) 161
Exercise Intolerance 162
Eyes (Swollen) 163
Failure to Thrive... 164
Family History of Breast Cancer 165
Family History of Coronary Disease 166
Family History of Diabetes....................................... 167
Family History of Gastrointestinal Malignancy 168
Fasciitis 169
Fatigue/Malaise 170
Fever 171
Fibrocystic Breast Disease....................................... 172
Fibroids (Uterine) 173
Fibromyalgia 174
Fibrositis.. 175
Flatulence 176
Flora- Restoration Post Antibiotic Therapy 177
Flu Shot Vaccine 178
Food Poisoning – Detoxification 179
Fracture.. 180
Frostbite 181
Fungal Infection 182
Furuncle/Carbuncle 183
Gallbladder Dysfunction... 184
Gangrene 185
Gas (Intestinal).. 186
Gastric Ulcer... 187
Gastroenteritis 188
Gastroesophageal Reflux 189
Gastroparesis... 190
Genital Warts 191
Gingivitis.. 192
Glaucoma.. 193
Glossitis 194
Glucose Intolerance... 195

Goiter..196
Gonorrhea...197
Gout 198
Graves' disease..199
Hair Loss (Non-Genetic) 200
Hangover...201
Hay Fever 202
Headache 203
Hearing Loss 204
Heavy Metal Toxicity...205
Hemiplegia/Hemiparesis due to Stroke 206
Hepatitis A 207
Hepatitis B 208
Hepatitis C 209
Herniated Intervertebral Disc...210
Herpes 211
Herpes Zoster...212
Herpes, Genital 213
HIV Disease..214
Hives...215
Hodgkins Disease 216
Hyperaldosteronism...217
Hypercholesterolemia 218
Hyperesthesia 219
Hyperhidrosos 220
Hyperlipidemia (Triglycerides}..221
Hypertension 222
Hyperthyroidism...223
Hyperventilation 224
Hypoglycemia 225
Hysterectomy 226
Ileitis...227
Immune Deficiency (Chronic)..228
Immune System Support..229
Impetigo..230
Impotence (Organic Erectile Dysfunction) 231
Incontinence Enuresis..232
Infection (Systemic) 233
Infertility (Female) 234
Infertility (Male)...235
Inflammation (Systemic) 236
Influenza w/ Respiratory Manifestations........................237
Insect Bite (venomous) 238
Insomnia...239
Intestinal Malabsorption..240
Irritable Bowel Syndrome (IBS) 241
Ischemic Bowel Disease...242
Itching (Pruritis) 243
Jaundice 244
Jock Itch...245

Joint pain (Multiple Sites)......246
Juvenile Arthritis 247
Kidney Detoxification......248
Kidney Infection 249
Labyrinthitis 250
Laryngitis......251
Leg Ulcers 252
Leukemia 253
Liver Disease (Chronic)......254
Lou Gehrig's Disease (ALS) 255
Low Blood Sugar 256
Lumbar Discitis......257
Lupus Erythematosis (SLE) 258
Lyme Disease 259
Lymph Nodes Swollen......260
Lymphadenitis 261
Lymphoma (Hodgkins) 262
Macular Degeneration 263
Malaria 264
Malignant Melanoma 265
Mastitis 266
Measles 267
Meniere's Syndrome 268
Meningitis 269
Menopausal Disorder 270
Menstrual Cramps (Dysmenorrhea) 271
Mental Retardation......272
Mercury Detoxification 273
Metastatic Carcinoma......274
Migraine......275
Mononucleosis 276
Mouth Sores......277
Multiple Myeloma......278
Multiple Sclerosis (MS) 279
Mumps 280
Myasthenia Gravis......281
Myocardial Infarction (non-acute) 282
Myocarditis 283
Myopathy 284
Narcolepsy 285
Nasal Polyp 286
Nausea......287
Nephritis......288
Neuralgia (Post-Herpetic) 289
Neurogenic Bladder 290
Neuromuscular Disorders......291
Night Sweats 292
Obesity 293
Optic Neuritis......294
Osteoarthritis......295

Osteomyelitis 296
Osteoporosis 297
Otitis Media 298
Ovaries (Infection) 399
Pain (Generalized)...300
Pain (pleuritic)...301
Palpitations 302
Pancreatitis (chronic)...303
Panic Disorder...304
Paraplegia 305
Parkinson's Disease..306
Pelvic Inflammatory Disease (PID) 307
Peptic Ulcers 308
Peripheral Vascular Disease 309
Pharyngitis (Sore Throat) 310
Pinkeye 311
Pleurisy..312
Pneumonia 313
Polio...314
Polymyalgia Rheumatica..315
Premenstrual Syndrome (PMS) 316
Prostatitis 317
Pruritis 318
Psoriasis 319
Psoriatic Arthritis 320
Pulmonary Fibrosis 321
Pulmonary Hypertension 322
Pyelonephritis 323
Rash 324
Raynaud's Syndrome..325
Reflex Sympathetic Dystrophy 326
Renal Failure Chronic 327
Restless Legs Syndrome 328
Retinitis 329
Rheumatoid Arthritis..330
Rosacea 331
Sarcoidosis..332
Seizure Disorder..333
Sepsis 334
Shingles 335
Shortness of Breath..336
Sick Sinus Syndrome 337
Sinusitis Chronic 338
Sjogren's Syndrome..339
SLE (Systemic Lupus Erythematosis)............................340
Sleep Apnea 341
Smallpox...342
Sore Throat 343
Spleen Infection 344
Splenomegaly 345

Staphylococcal Food Poisoning (Detoxification) 346
Stomach Problems..347
Stomatitis 348
Strep Throat (Pharyngitis)..349
Stress (Physical or Emotional) 350
Sugar Craving 351
Surgery (During Recovery) 352
Systemic Lupus Erythematosis (SLE)............................353
Temporal Arteritis 354
Tension Headache (Chronic) 355
Thrombocytopenia..356
Thyroiditis (Acute) 357
Tissue Trauma 358
Tobacco Dependence 359
Tonsillitis 360
Tonsils (Swollen) 361
Ulcerative Colitis 362
Ulcers- Diabetic...363
Urethritis 364
Urinary Tract Infection (UTI) 365
Uterine Fibroids 366
Vaginitis/Vulvitis (Candida)..367
Varicella (Chickenpox) 368
Vasculitis 369
Venereal Disease 370
Vertigo (Dizziness) 371
Viral Infection 372
Warts 373

Part III: Recommendations for Conditions Not Listed........375

Recommendations for Conditions Not Listed 377

Part IV: Appendix 379

Appendix 1: Product Definitions Nutritional Daily Menu 381
Appendix 2: Resources 382

PART I: Introduction

"There is no such thing as a miracle which violates natural law. There are only occurrences which violate our limited knowledge of natural law."
-St. Augustine

2

Read This First - How To Use This Book:

This is a "how-to" book on the use of specific nutrients and meridian point therapy. This book is meant to be used by those wishing direction in healing the body utilizing fundamental cell communication molecules – beginning with the glyconutrient class as well as supporting the body with meridian system support – otherwise known as Glyco-Meridian Therapy™.

We have alphabetically listed over 350 specific health challenges by name and their related Glyco-Meridian protocols. These support protocols are neither medical treatment nor advice for these conditions. Always consult your own medical professional for specific medical conditions. The nutritional ingredients listed under the nutritional menu heading are listed as generic products. The following terms are utilized: Glyco, Phyto, Pre-Hormone, Essentials or Catablend. You then must determine what types of products and serving sizes are needed for your specific health challenge. At this point turn to the Product Definitions for Nutritional Daily Menu located in appendix 1 (page 381). If you suffer from multiple conditions, prioritize your number one complaint and address that first.

Abbreviations used in Part II of the conditions section are as follows: tsp indicates teaspoon; tabs indicate tablets.

The recommended serving sizes in this book are for adults. Servings for children less than 12 years of age can be found by contacting the corporate office of the company noted in appendix 1.

The chapter entitled, "Rules for Meridian Point Stimulation", presents an overview on how to begin using the meridian system as an adjunct to nutrient recommendation. Many of these techniques have been utilized for thousands of years and many are based upon the clinical successes of the authors.

If your condition is not listed, refer to Part III, entitled "Summary of General Recommendations for Conditions Not Listed".

Appendix 2 contains an extensive list of recommended products and resources. The criteria for choosing products are based upon the authors clinical experience while some of the recommendations are made on the basis of analyzing current scientific principals.

3

A Personal Message from Dr. Schlachter

You will not heal by taking drugs. Your health and healing is determined by how well you eat. Our food supply is lacking appropriate nutrients and this cannot be helped by synthetic additives. The only rational approach to health is to take food based nutrients in supplemental form. It is your responsibility to decide which nutrients are best for you and your family.

As you make the elementary changes in your diet that have been addressed in this book, your body will undergo a change. When your body assimilates these nutrients you will experience an increased sense of well-being. Other times, this change is preceded by a reaction of the body ridding itself of toxins and changing the way cells communicate. Some call this a "cleansing crisis", "correcting crisis" or "toxic reaction". Probably the best way to think about this is to remember what the body initially goes through when you begin an exercise regimen after a long period of inactivity. You often experience aches and pains as your body adjusts. The same process holds true when the body has been in a nutritionally "inactive" state.

One of the first things you notice when you optimize your nutrition is that you do not tire so easily. You begin experiencing more sustained energy, feel less fatigued, enjoy an increased sense of well-being and experience more emotional strength. People around you will begin to notice that the little things do not bother you as they once did. Symptoms from disease process generally improve over weeks to months. As you improve, your dependency on pharmaceuticals will lessen. For this reason, close contact with your health care provider is needed to closely monitor the need for and tapering of your medications.

Many of you who are sick are wondering – will I get better if I use the protocols from this book? Virtually everyone who improves their nutrition will experience a positive change in their health. This improvement may occur quickly or over months. In my practice there has been no symptom, no problem, no complaint, no disease, no syndrome, in or out of the hospital, in or out of the intensive care unit that has not been helped by these nutrient protocols.

Dr. Schlachter

A Personal Message from Dr. Aristotle

Research has shown that in addition to the arteries, veins, lymphatics and nerves, there exists a bioelectric energetic conduit known as the meridian system. These acupuncture meridians conduct energy throughout the entire body affecting structure, function and emotion. An ancient translation taught to first year students of Eastern Medicine is the following:

"A Meridian Affects Where It Courses Through and To..."

Types of health problems addressed through Meridian Point Therapy™ may include, but are not limited to, physical pain, chronic and acute illness, hormonal changes, emotional difficulty, structural changes, fatigue, etc.

A few causes of blocked meridians include:
-Scar tissue as a result of surgery or injury
-Emotional and environmental stresses
-Physical stress and trauma
-Poor diet
-Environmental toxins

Along each meridian there are specific meridian points. Over the centuries these points are known to specifically affect certain conditions. If a meridian becomes blocked then illness occurs. It is that simple. While treating meridian imbalances, practitioners stimulate specific points on each meridian to assist in the "unlocking" of stagnant electrical energy. This restoration process removes energy blockages, resumes balance and functioning of the body's internal organs and structures.

Methods of stimulating these points will vary. At times, acupressure is used in which the points are rubbed with the fingers or tapped with a non-invasive hand held instrument called a *teishein* (tay-sheen). Light stimulation, such as a soft laser (one of my favorites), may also be applied as well as a variety of massage techniques. This book outlines those unique points specific to each health challenge and offers a starting point and foundation for those individuals suffering from illness.

Many of the points listed in this book are not recorded in any textbook. During my research tour throughout hospitals within The People's Republic of China, a practitioner of the healing arts personally gave them to me. These are treasured points that have been handed down from generation to generation throughout the centuries from families of Asian decent.

This is the first time I am sharing them in book form.

They are known as "Miracle Points".

Dr. Aristotle

Emergency and Maintenance Menu Definitions

In Part II: Conditions, we list specific problems and their recommended daily servings ("RDS"). In this section, the following terms are used and their definitions and importance to health issues are listed below.

Glyco:
Glyconutrients – form the basic cellular language of all cells; proper amounts allow cells to communicate properly. These types of nutrients improve the immune system and the antioxidant levels inside the cells. Examples of immune system dysfunction include allergies, cancer, lupus, asthma and slow wound healing.

Phyto:
Phytonutrients - there are over 10,000 in number known to date. Phytonutrients are found in vegetables and fruits. Phytonutrients are pivotal in heart disease prevention and cancer fighting activity. Phytonutrients include free radical scavengers and anti-oxidants. They have synergistic duties with the glyconutrients.

Pre-Hormone:
Phytosterols – Proper cellular functioning requires molecules that provide proper endocrine function. This includes the more than seventy different hormones that help regulate the body. Examples include DHEA, progesterone, testosterone etc. Significant benefit can be seen with ingestion of a standardized wild yam (Beta Sitosterol Complex).

Essentials and Catablend:
Mineral and Vitamins (Classical Nutrition) – Of utmost importance, these minerals and vitamins must be ingested in a form as close to food as possible and include such terms as food-form or food matrix vitamins. Also, completion of a Dietary Needs Assessment is highly recommended in order to identify which combination of foods (proteins, fats, and carbohydrates) you should ingest. There are two types of minerals, vitamins and antioxidants complexes recommended. Essentials, which contain the standard or basic amounts of minerals, vitamins and anti-oxidants. Catablend is our term for a vitamin, mineral and anti-oxidant complex that has more of the essential nutrients and anti-oxidants and is typically needed for more severe symptoms or medical problems.

Healing Reactions (Cell Memory and Retracing)

In a small number of people, several transient reactions may occur while the body attempts to physiologically balance the body chemistry and revitalize the immune system through the support of cellular communication via Glyco-Meridian Therapy™ . The longer the deficiencies have existed, the more prevalent the response is likely to be. This response is known as retracing. During retracing, the cells release a type of memory that contains the information that eventually led up to your current disease state. During this process you may experience symptoms of prior illness such as fever, rash, hives, excessive gas, runny nose, headaches, insomnia, increased thirst, weakness, lethargy, loss of appetite, nausea, diarrhea, fever blisters, dry mouth, canker sores, constipation, dizziness, nervousness, as well as various body aches and pains. Please understand that these are corrective reactions.

When you apply Glyco-Meridian Therapy, you can be assured your body is making positive changes toward an improved state of health. Understand that these short-term reactions are part of the healing process. This is a small price to pay for long-lasting health benefits.

Tips To Handle Healing Reactions

1. Drink plenty of water. This amount should be half of your body weight in ounces per day. For example, if you weigh 100 pounds then you should drink 50 oz. per day. The quality of the water is important, therefore, non-carbonated water in glass bottle is ideal (plastic containers leach polycarbons into the water). Drinking water will help flush out the toxins and contribute to the natural cleansing of the organ systems. If you have a heart or kidney problem, please check with your healthcare provider before embarking on this amount of water.

2. Increase your intake of fruits, vegetables, and bran from cereals. This can help accelerate the removal of toxins of any type.

3. Include an activity component in your daily routine. Walking or bicycling for 15 minutes a day is a good place to start.

4. Apply the meridian points during your detoxification and healing process. As symptoms of healing reactions appear, simply stimulate the points indicated on the meridian charts that are specific to your condition.

5. When bathing, be sure to use a loofa, a bath brush or a coarse sponge to assist in the cleansing of your skin.

6. If the healing reaction is too strong for you to tolerate, you can reduce or even discontinue the supplements for a couple of days, and then gradually increase to the recommended amounts. This routine may need to be repeated depending on the depleted condition of your body and the amount of repair needed at the cellular level.

What To Do About Specific Diseases?

If you are taking medications for a disease and you improve your nutrition, your requirements for medications will invariably diminish. It is important that you inform your health care provider that you will need less medication over time.

Specific "menus" for health issues and diseases are included in this book. It is important to note that these suggestions are not recommendations for therapy and do not substitute for diagnosis and treatment by your own personal health care provider. For conditions not listed, general guidelines are listed in Part III, "Recommendations for Conditions Not Listed".

These recommendations are targets or goals. Work up to larger amounts by starting 1/4 teaspoon 2 x day and increase every 3 to 7 days to the target amount. In general, when you are using symptoms as an indicator for taking more (or less) product, make changes in 1 to 4 week intervals. It may take 3 to 6 months for some to change their body's functioning; for others, it may take 1 to 2 years.

Once you experience the desired effect, it will be possible to reduce the amounts by following the same rules as above. Once you begin Glyco-Meridian Therapy™, it's always up to you how long you want to be healthy and free of disease.

Glyco-Meridian Therapy™ in the Hospital Environment

A hospital environment is an incredibly important setting to use Glyco-Meridian protocols. There are various rules and regulations concerning the use of nutritional supplements at some institutions in the United States. The common denominator is that supplements require the authorization by the attending physician. The reasoning for this is that drug effects and interactions need to be monitored closely. Side effects are not a problem with meridian therapy and meridian applications will not interfere with any medication. Generally speaking, if the physician agrees to the use of supplements, a waiver of responsibility may have to be signed by the patient or by the family member. Please remember it is your responsibility to inquire about other options and other treatment protocols with your doctor.

There have been a number of cases across the country where the attending staff or the hospital prohibited the use of natural whole food supplements. Under these conditions, legal action may be needed to ensure that nutrients are given. In reference to the meridian point stimulation, there are no known regulations that prohibit its use. In fact, many hospitals now incorporate the principals of meridian therapy. One of these is commonly known as acupuncture.

Some hospitals will not allow supplements to be given by family members. This results in diminished nutrition. Because this is often problematic, as a family member or patient, this is likely to cause you significant concern. You may be able to set up a meeting with the doctor, head nurse, or the nurse caring for your loved one. Ask them how to make sure the food supplements are administered and offer your help as well. Additionally, make sure that there is always product available for the nurses and that the directions for dosages are very clear. Once again, legal action may be necessary if the hospital does not cooperate.

The patient in the intensive care unit (ICU) requires unique and special attention. The patient is often not able to take in any food or liquid by mouth and a feeding tube is inserted via the nose into the stomach. If long term feeding is required with a stomach tube, a surgical tube called a "PEG tube" is used. There are some instances where these tubes are not utilized and patients are fed hospital supplied nutrition via an intravenous route. At the time of this writing there are no intravenous products available for the glyconutrients.

To use the naso-gastric tube (also termed NG tube) or a PEG tube, it is important that the mixture of nutrients is thin enough to pass through the tube without plugging it. The typical mixture is 1 tablespoon of glyconutrient powder with 6 to 8 oz. of spring bottled water or tube feeding solution. Make sure the solution is free of any clumps. The mixture is then given through the tube and natural spring water is flushed through the tube to clear the mixture (helps to prevent clogging). Sometimes the number of nursing staff is often suboptimal, too busy to follow protocols or simply forget to administer the glyconutrients. Under these circumstances it may help to administer larger amounts less frequently as opposed to, say, a teaspoon every hour.

If a patient is in the intensive care unit, the one teaspoon every hour can be done fairly easily, as the patient is generally assigned a nurse that cares for a total of one or two patients. Remember, it will be your responsibility to monitor the administration of nutrients.

When implementing meridian point stimulation, apply at least three (3) times a day in the ICU. Points should be stimulated with either finger point pressure, soft laser or tei shein application. These are all non-invasive and application is simple. Please refer to rules for meridian point stimulation on the following page.

Rules for Meridian Point Stimulation

The meridian points in this book are only shown for one half the body (unilateral) to simplify the diagram. The body has points on both sides of the body and need to be stimulated. For example: a point shown on the left leg will also exist on the right leg and needs stimulation; a point on the right lower abdomen also exist on the opposite side (mirror image) and needs to be stimulated. Points that are midline have no duplicate (mirror image) points. Please note, many times when a meridian point is in need of therapeutic application, the point will be sore to the touch. You may need to "browse" around the area of the point to locate the tender spot.

Scar tissue on the body will inhibit the functioning of the meridian system. If you or a loved one is suffering from a health condition it is the recommendation of these authors to stimulate scar tissue. This includes scars from past surgeries over one month and injuries. Soft laser application can be started three days after surgery. Acceptable methods of general scar tissue stimulation are soft laser, gentle massage or teishein. Stimulate old scars at least once a day for 30 seconds.

Finger pressure: Direct finger pressure is applied to the skin directly on the meridian point. Use firm pressure without causing discomfort. Massage the meridian point 30 to 45 seconds. Perform in a crisis situation 3 times a day. For chronic problems, perform once a day.

Teishein (*tay-sheen*): Lightly tap the meridian point as shown in the diagram 20 times. The non-invasive teishein is one of the classic pressure needles. Its use is worldwide, found in clinics, hospitals and research institutes. It is a favorite of health care practitioners. Perform in a crisis situation 3 times a day. For chronic problems, perform once a day.

Soft laser: Hold the laser tip (the end of the laser) approximately ½ to 1 inch from the meridian point or desired area. Stimulate with the laser 30 seconds to 1 minute per point. A clockwise circular motion is recommended. Perform in a crisis situation 3 times a day. For chronic problems, perform once a day.

PART II: Conditions

13

Abdominal Pain, General

Emergency Nutritional Daily Menu	Maintenance Nutritional Daily Menu
Glyco: 3 tsp Phyto: 1/2 tsp Pre-Hormone: 3 tabs Essentials: 4 tabs	Glyco: 1 tsp Phyto: 1/2 tsp Pre-Hormone: 3 tabs Essentials: 4 tabs

see appendix for product definitions

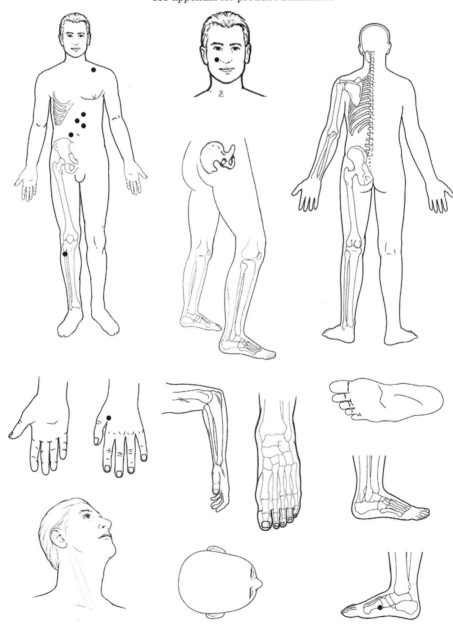

14

Abscess, Skin

Emergency Nutritional Daily Menu	Maintenance Nutritional Daily Menu
Glyco: 2 tsp Phyto: 1/2 tsp Pre-Hormone: 3 tabs Essentials: 4 tabs	Glyco: 1 tsp Phyto: 1/2 tsp Pre-Hormone: 3 tabs Essentials: 4 tabs

see appendix for product definitions

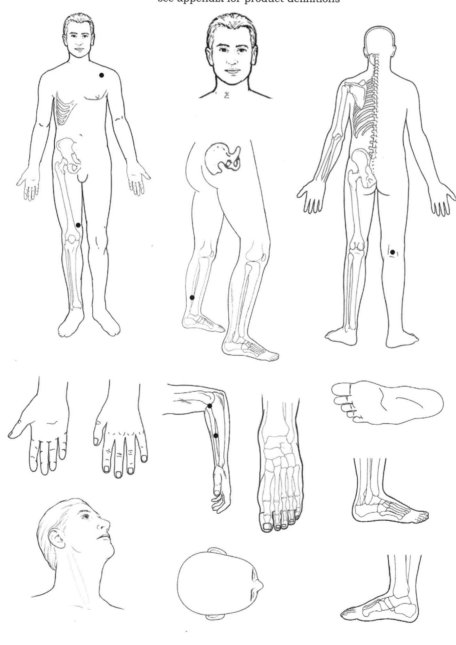

Acne
(apply soft laser to affected areas)

Emergency Nutritional Daily Menu	Maintenance Nutritional Daily Menu
Glyco: 2 tsp Phyto: 1/2 tsp Pre-Hormone: 3 tabs Essentials: 4 tabs	Glyco: 1 tsp Phyto: 1/2 tsp Pre-Hormone: 3 tabs Essentials: 4 tabs

see appendix for product definitions

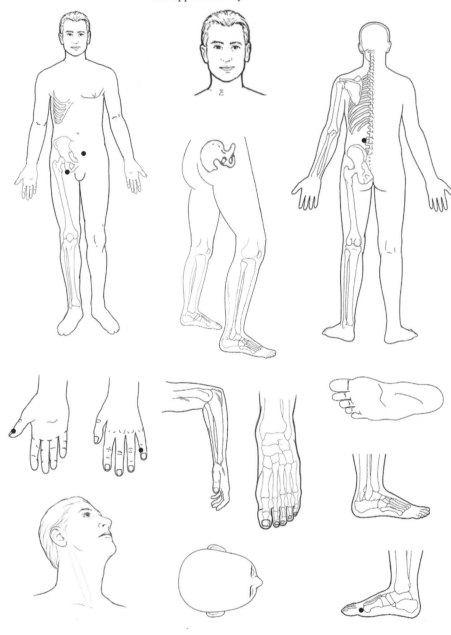

Actinic Keratosis

Emergency Nutritional Daily Menu	Maintenance Nutritional Daily Menu
Glyco: 2 tsp Phyto: 1/2 tsp Pre-Hormone: 3 tabs Cata-Blend: 4 tabs	Glyco: 1 tsp Phyto: 1/2 tsp Pre-Hormone: 3 tabs Cata-Blend: 4 tabs

see appendix for product definitions

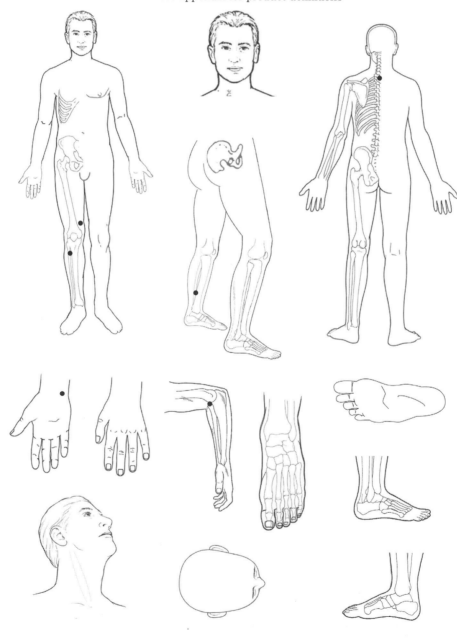

ADD w/Hyperactivity

Emergency Nutritional Daily Menu	Maintenance Nutritional Daily Menu
Glyco: 3 tsp Phyto: 1/2 tsp Pre-Hormone: 3 tabs Cata-Blend: 4 tabs	Glyco: 1 tsp Phyto: 1/2 tsp Pre-Hormone: 3 tabs Cata-Blend: 4 tabs

see appendix for product definitions

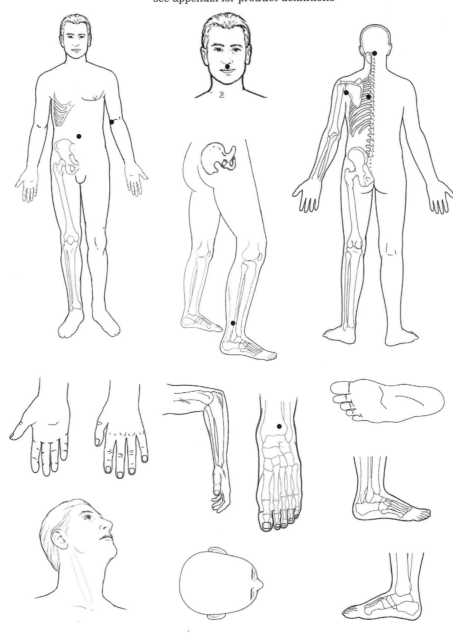

Addiction

Emergency Nutritional Daily Menu	Maintenance Nutritional Daily Menu
Glyco: 3 tsp Phyto: 1/2 tsp Pre-Hormone: 3 tabs Cata-Blend: 6 tabs	Glyco: 2 tsp Phyto: 1/2 tsp Pre-Hormone: 3 tabs Cata-Blend: 6 tabs

see appendix for product definitions

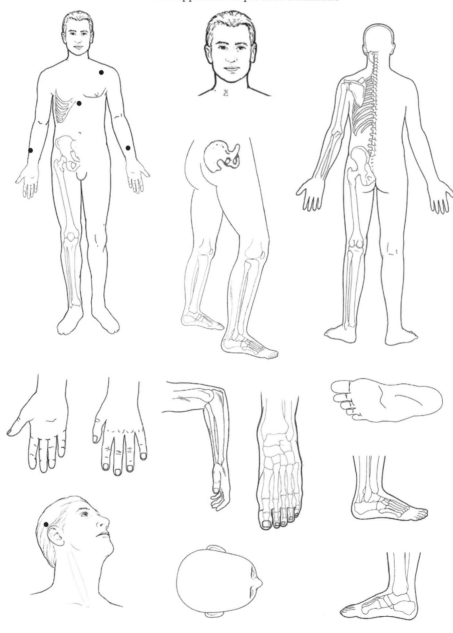

19

Adrenal Exhaustion

Emergency Nutritional Daily Menu	Maintenance Nutritional Daily Menu
Glyco: 4 tsp Phyto: 2 tsp Pre-Hormone: 6 tabs Cata-Blend: 6 tabs	Glyco: 2 tsp Phyto: 1 tsp Pre-Hormone: 3 tabs Cata-Blend: 4 tabs

see appendix for product definitions

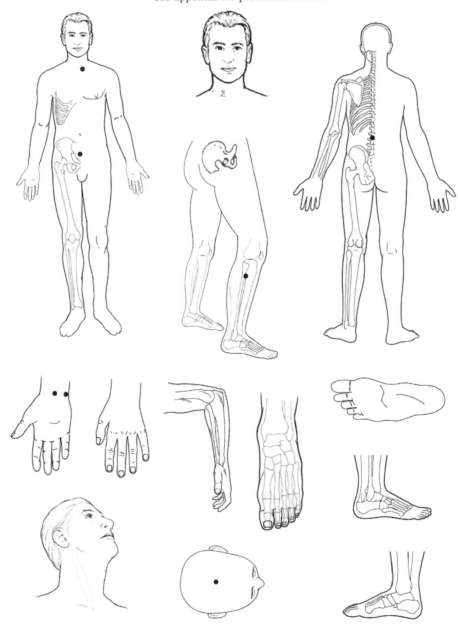

Adrenal Insufficiency (Addison's Disease)

Emergency Nutritional Daily Menu	Maintenance Nutritional Daily Menu
Glyco: 4 tsp Phyto: 2 tsp Pre-Hormone: 6 tabs Cata-Blend: 4 tabs	Glyco: 2 tsp Phyto: 1 tsp Pre-Hormone: 3 tabs Cata-Blend: 4 tabs

see appendix for product definitions

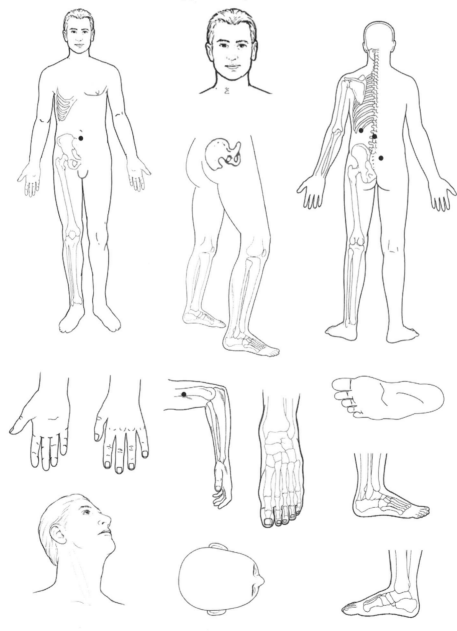

Adult Respiratory Distress Syndrome (ARDS)

Emergency Nutritional Daily Menu	Maintenance Nutritional Daily Menu
Glyco: 12 tsp Phyto: 3 tsp Pre-Hormone: 3 tabs Cata-Blend: 6 tabs	Glyco: 3 tsp Phyto: 1 tsp Pre-Hormone: 3 tabs Cata-Blend: 4 tabs

see appendix for product definitions

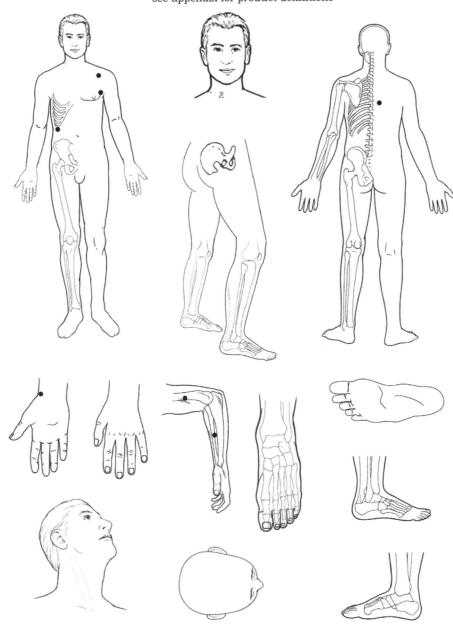

22

AIDS

Emergency Nutritional Daily Menu	Maintenance Nutritional Daily Menu
Glyco: 12 tsp Phyto: 4 tsp Pre-Hormone: 6 tabs Cata-Blend: 6 tabs	Glyco: 3 tsp Phyto: 2 tsp Pre-Hormone: 3 tabs Cata-Blend: 6 tabs

see appendix for product definitions

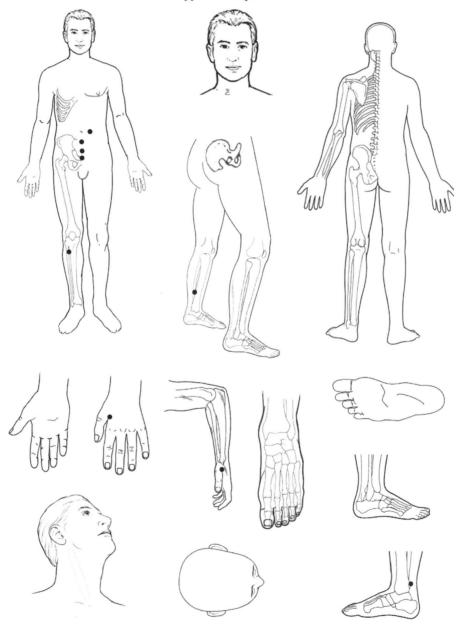

Alcohol Abuse

Emergency Nutritional Daily Menu	Maintenance Nutritional Daily Menu
Glyco: 6 tsp Phyto: 2 tsp Pre-Hormone: 6 tabs Cata-Blend: 4 tabs	Glyco: 2 tsp Phyto: 1 tsp Pre-Hormone: 4 tabs Cata-Blend: 4 tabs

see appendix for product definitions

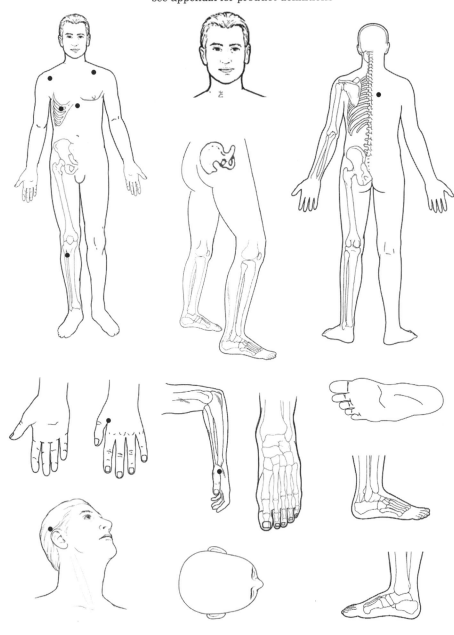

Allergic Rhinitis

Emergency Nutritional Daily Menu	Maintenance Nutritional Daily Menu
Glyco: 3 tsp Phyto: 1/2 tsp Pre-Hormone: 3 tabs Essentials: 4 tabs	Glyco: 1 tsp Phyto: 1/2 tsp Pre-Hormone: 3 tabs Essentials: 4 tabs

see appendix for product definitions

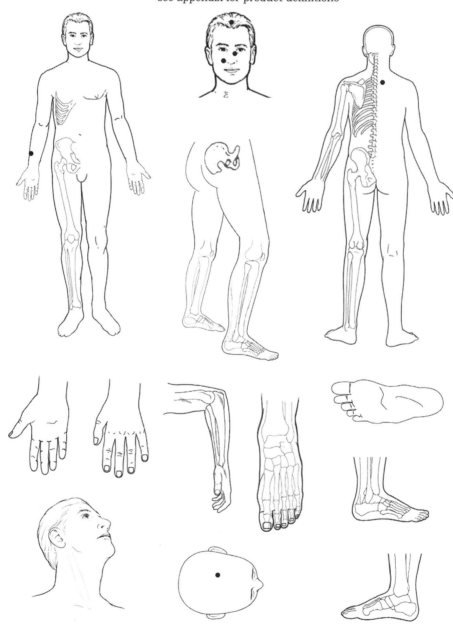

Allergy

Emergency Nutritional Daily Menu	Maintenance Nutritional Daily Menu
Glyco: 3 tsp Phyto: 1/2 tsp Pre-Hormone: 3 tabs Essentials: 4 tabs	Glyco: 1 tsp Phyto: 1/2 tsp Pre-Hormone: 3 tabs Essentials: 4 tabs

see appendix for product definitions

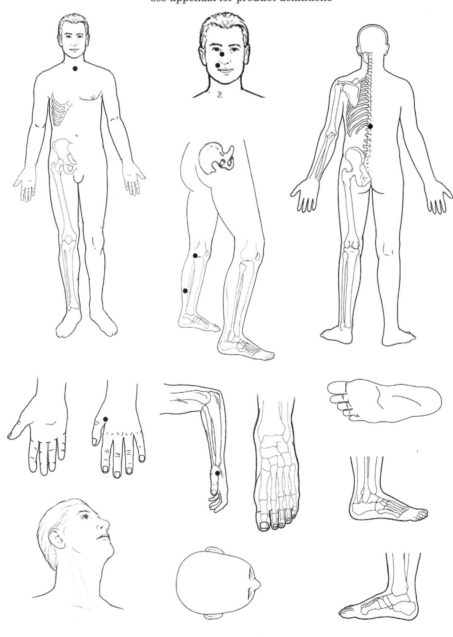

26

Alopecia

Emergency Nutritional Daily Menu	Maintenance Nutritional Daily Menu
Glyco: 3 tsp Phyto: 2 tsp Pre-Hormone: 6 tabs Essentials: 4 tabs	Glyco: 1 tsp Phyto: 1/2 tsp Pre-Hormone: 3 tabs Essentials: 4 tabs

see appendix for product definitions

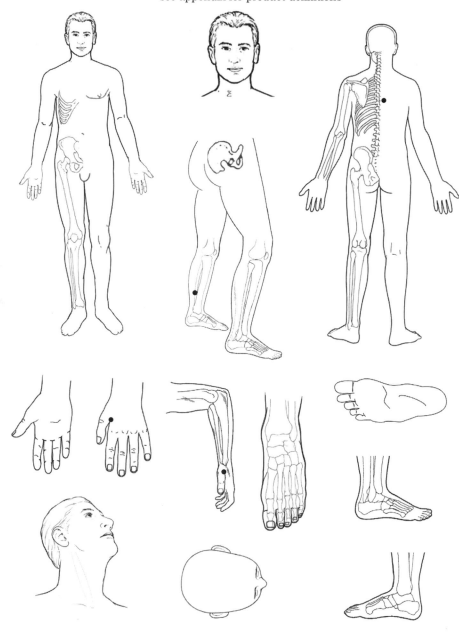

ALS (Amyotrophic Lateral Sclerosis)

Emergency Nutritional Daily Menu	Maintenance Nutritional Daily Menu
Glyco: 12 tsp Phyto: 2 tsp Pre-Hormone: 6 tabs Cata-Blend: 6 tabs	Glyco: 6 tsp Phyto: 2 tsp Pre-Hormone: 4 tabs Cata-Blend: 6 tabs

see appendix for product definitions

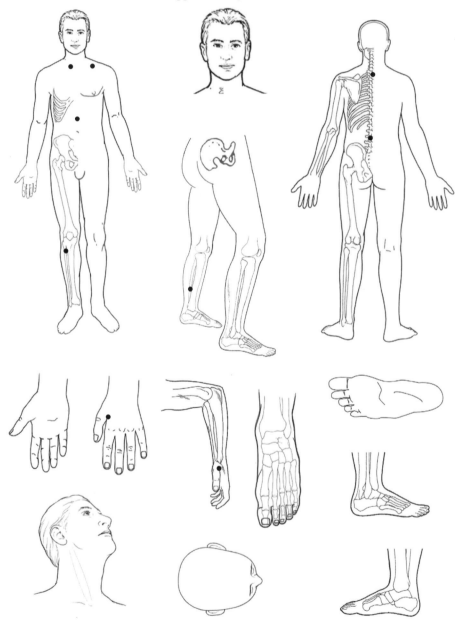

Alzheimer's (Dementia)

Emergency Nutritional Daily Menu	Maintenance Nutritional Daily Menu
Glyco: 12 tsp Phyto: 2 tsp Pre-Hormone: 6 tabs Cata-Blend: 6 tabs	Glyco: 6 tsp Phyto: 2 tsp Pre-Hormone: 6 tabs Cata-Blend: 6 tabs

see appendix for product definitions

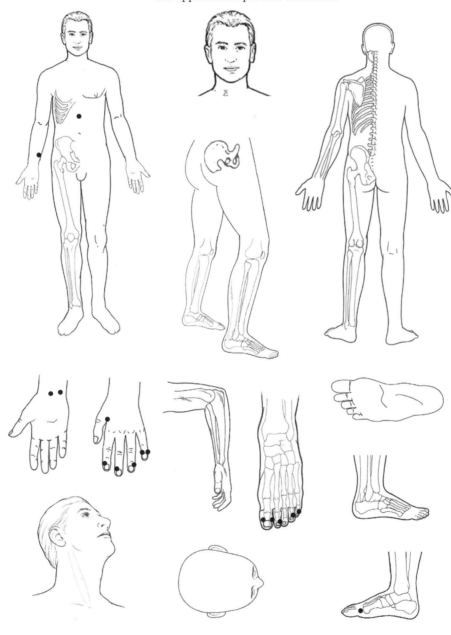

Amalgam Toxicity

Emergency Nutritional Daily Menu	Maintenance Nutritional Daily Menu
Glyco: 6 tsp Phyto: 2 tsp Pre-Hormone: 3 tabs Cata-Blend: 6 tabs	Glyco: 2 tsp Phyto: 1/2 tsp Pre-Hormone: 3 tabs Cata-Blend: 6 tabs

see appendix for product definitions

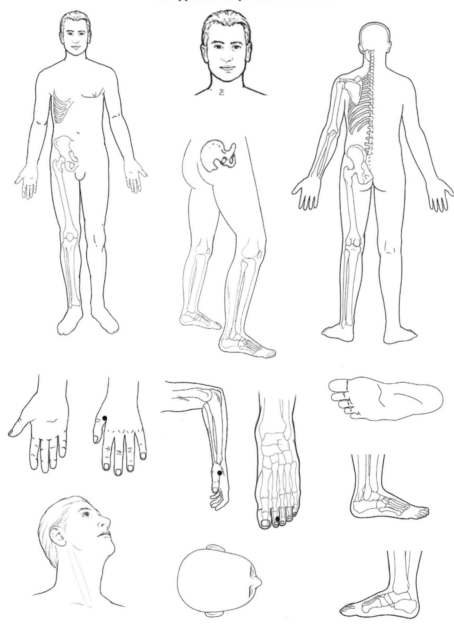

30

Amenorrhea

Emergency Nutritional Daily Menu	Maintenance Nutritional Daily Menu
Glyco: 3 tsp Phyto: 1 tsp Pre-Hormone: 6 tabs Cata-Blend: 4 tabs	Glyco: 2 tsp Phyto: 1/2 tsp Pre-Hormone: 4 tabs Cata-Blend: 4 tabs

see appendix for product definitions

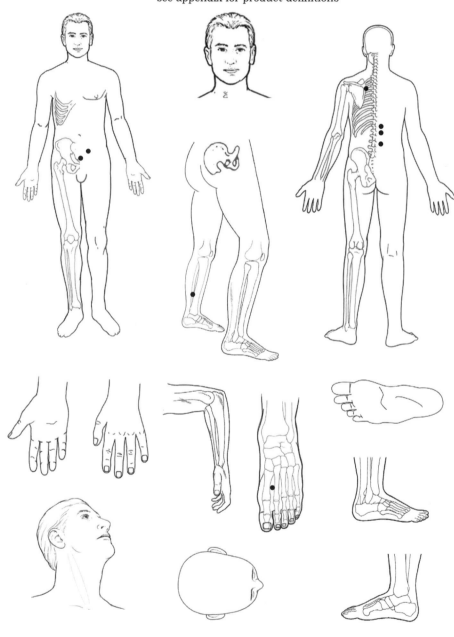

Amyotrophic Lateral Sclerosis (ALS)

Emergency Nutritional Daily Menu	Maintenance Nutritional Daily Menu
Glyco: 12 tsp Phyto: 2 tsp Pre-Hormone: 6 tabs Cata-Blend: 6 tabs	Glyco: 6 tsp Phyto: 2 tsp Pre-Hormone: 4 tabs Cata-Blend: 6 tabs

see appendix for product definitions

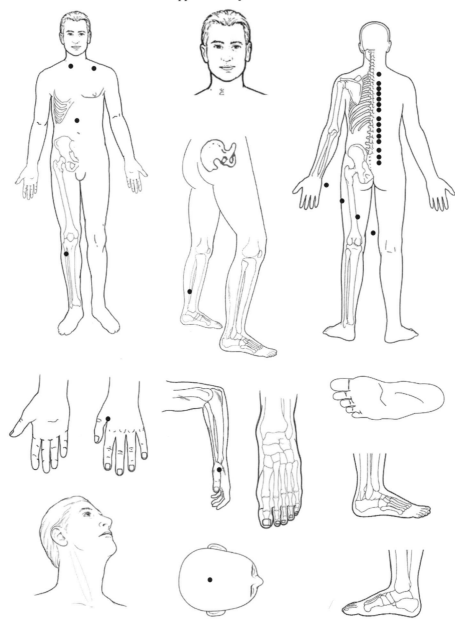

32

Anemia

Emergency Nutritional Daily Menu	Maintenance Nutritional Daily Menu
Glyco: 3 tsp Phyto: 1 tsp Pre-Hormone: 3 tabs Essentials: 4 tabs	Glyco: 2 tsp Phyto: 1 tsp Pre-Hormone: 3 tabs Essentials: 4 tabs

see appendix for product definitions

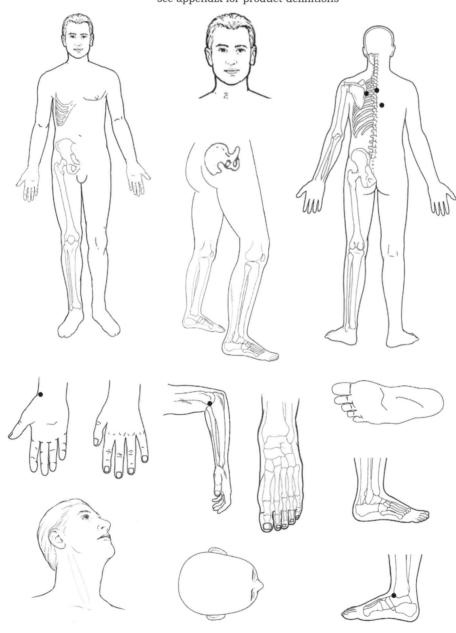

Anemia, Sickle Cell

Emergency Nutritional Daily Menu	Maintenance Nutritional Daily Menu
Glyco: 3 tsp Phyto: 1 tsp Pre-Hormone: 3 tabs Essentials: 4 tabs	Glyco: 2 tsp Phyto: 1 tsp Pre-Hormone: 3 tabs Essentials: 4 tabs

see appendix for product definitions

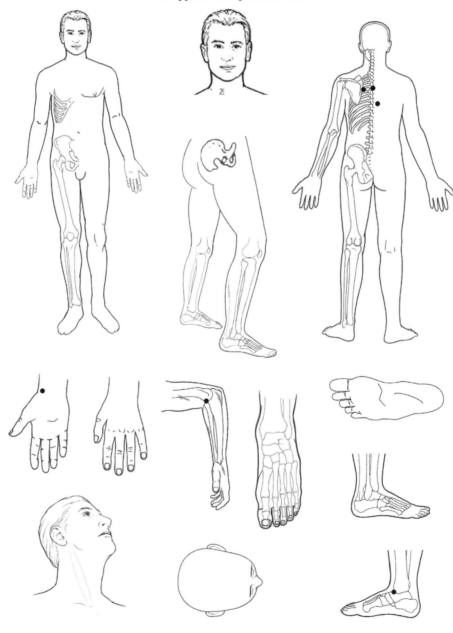

Aneurysm (Aortic)

Emergency Nutritional Daily Menu	Maintenance Nutritional Daily Menu
Glyco: 6 tsp Phyto: 3 tsp Pre-Hormone: 4 tabs Essentials: 4 tabs	Glyco: 3 tsp Phyto: 1 tsp Pre-Hormone: 3 tabs Essentials: 4 tabs

see appendix for product definitions

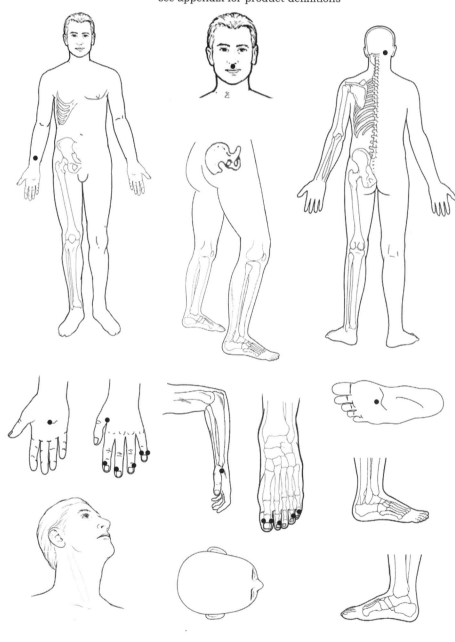

Angina Pectoris

Emergency Nutritional Daily Menu	Maintenance Nutritional Daily Menu
Glyco: 6 tsp Phyto: 1 tsp Pre-Hormone: 4 tabs Cata-Blend: 6 tabs	Glyco: 2 tsp Phyto: 1 tsp Pre-Hormone: 3 tabs Cata-Blend: 6 tabs

see appendix for product definitions

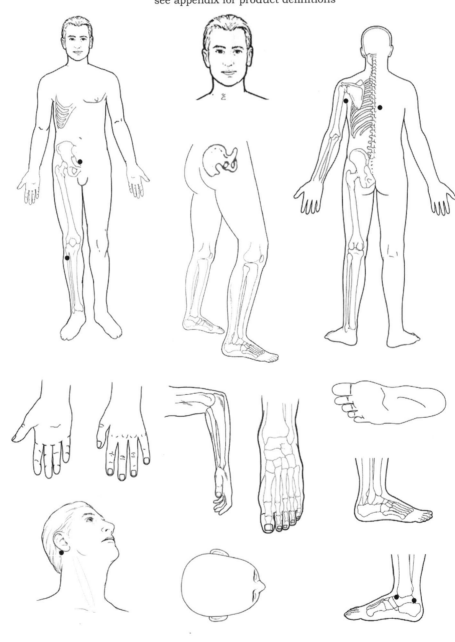

Angioneurotic Edema

Emergency Nutritional Daily Menu	Maintenance Nutritional Daily Menu
Glyco: 6 tsp Phyto: 1 tsp Pre-Hormone: 4 tabs Cata-Blend: 6 tabs	Glyco: 2 tsp Phyto: 1 tsp Pre-Hormone: 3 tabs Cata-Blend: 4 tabs

see appendix for product definitions

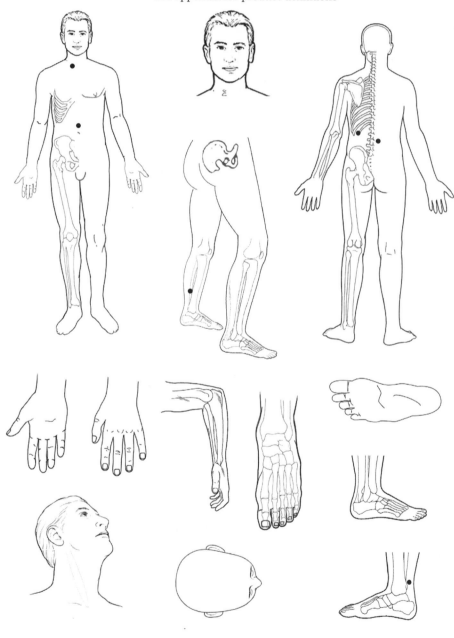

Ankylosing Spondylitis (AS)

Emergency Nutritional Daily Menu	Maintenance Nutritional Daily Menu
Glyco: 2 tsp Phyto: 1/2 tsp Pre-Hormone: 6 tabs Essentials: 4 tabs	Glyco: 2 tsp Phyto: 1/2 tsp Pre-Hormone: 3 tabs Essentials: 4 tabs

see appendix for product definitions

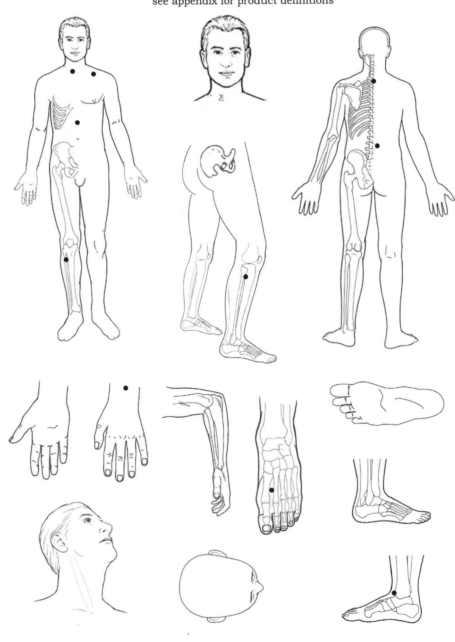

38

Anorexia

Emergency Nutritional Daily Menu	Maintenance Nutritional Daily Menu
Glyco: 4 tsp Phyto: 2 tsp Pre-Hormone: 6 tabs Essentials: 4 tabs	Glyco: 2 tsp Phyto: 1 tsp Pre-Hormone: 4 tabs Essentials: 4 tabs

see appendix for product definitions

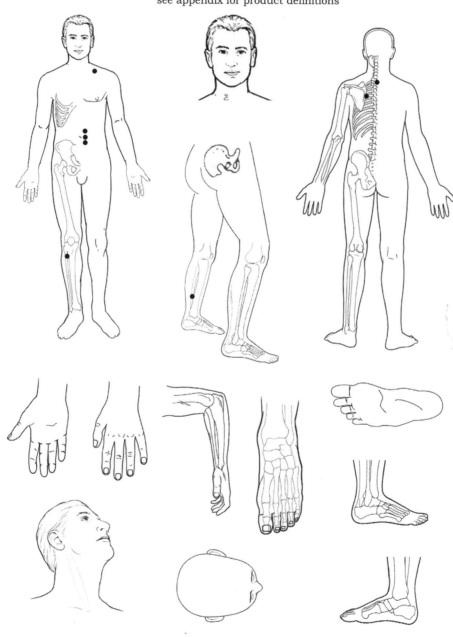

39

Anorexia Nervosa

Emergency Nutritional Daily Menu	Maintenance Nutritional Daily Menu
Glyco: 6 tsp Phyto: 2 tsp Pre-Hormone: 6 tabs Essentials: 4 tabs	Glyco: 2 tsp Phyto: 1 tsp Pre-Hormone: 4 tabs Essentials: 4 tabs

see appendix for product definitions

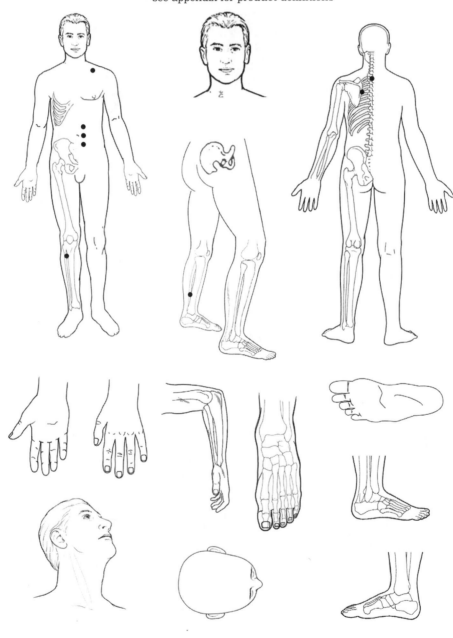

Antihistamine

Emergency Nutritional Daily Menu	Maintenance Nutritional Daily Menu
Glyco: 2 tsp Phyto: 1 tsp Pre-Hormone: 4 tabs Essentials: 4 tabs	Glyco: 1 tsp Phyto: 1/2 tsp Pre-Hormone: 3 tabs Essentials: 4 tabs

see appendix for product definitions

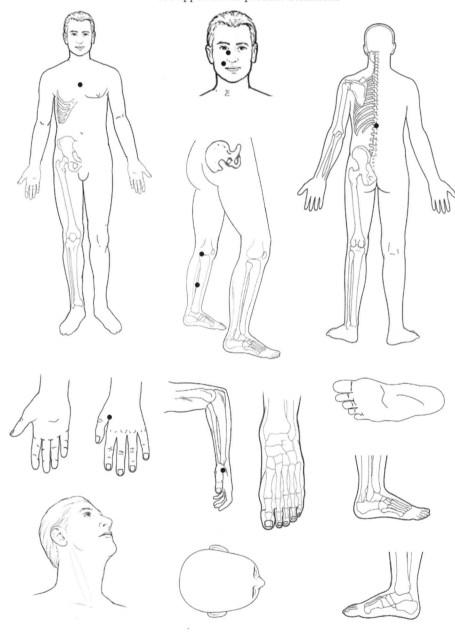

Anxiety State

Emergency Nutritional Daily Menu	Maintenance Nutritional Daily Menu
Glyco: 3 tsp Phyto: 1 tsp Pre-Hormone: 6 tabs Essentials: 4 tabs	Glyco: 1 tsp Phyto: 1/2 tsp Pre-Hormone: 3 tabs Essentials: 4 tabs

see appendix for product definitions

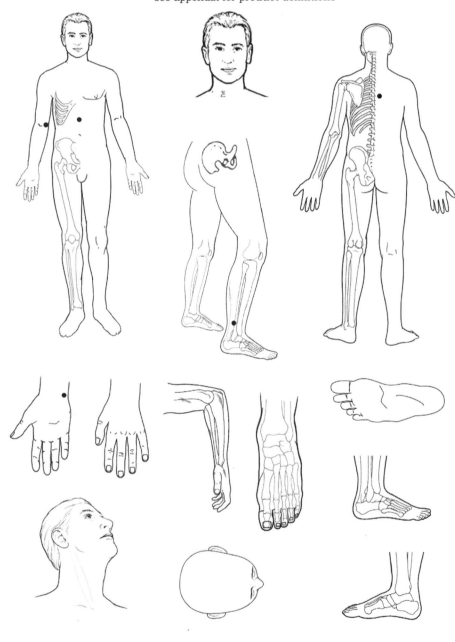

Aphthous Ulcer (Canker Sore)

Emergency Nutritional Daily Menu	Maintenance Nutritional Daily Menu
Glyco: 3 tsp Phyto: 1/2 tsp Pre-Hormone: 4 tabs Essentials: 4 tabs	Glyco: 1 tsp Phyto: 1/2 tsp Pre-Hormone: 3 tabs Essentials: 4 tabs

see appendix for product definitions

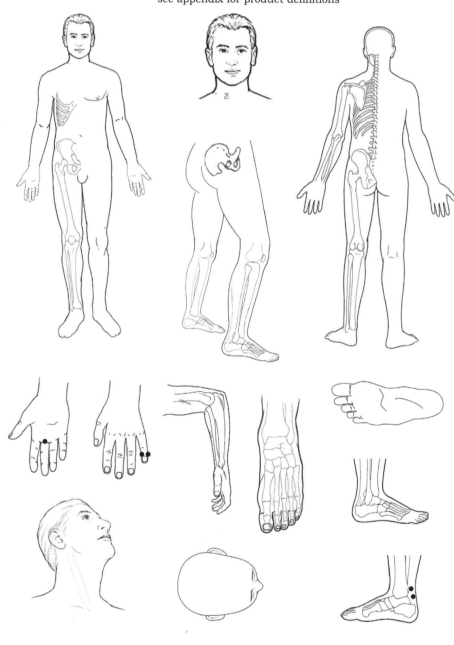

43

Arrhythmia

Emergency Nutritional Daily Menu	Maintenance Nutritional Daily Menu
Glyco: 6 tsp Phyto: 2 tsp Pre-Hormone: 4 tabs Cata-Blend: 6 tabs	Glyco: 2 tsp Phyto: 1 tsp Pre-Hormone: 3 tabs Cata-Blend: 6 tabs

see appendix for product definitions

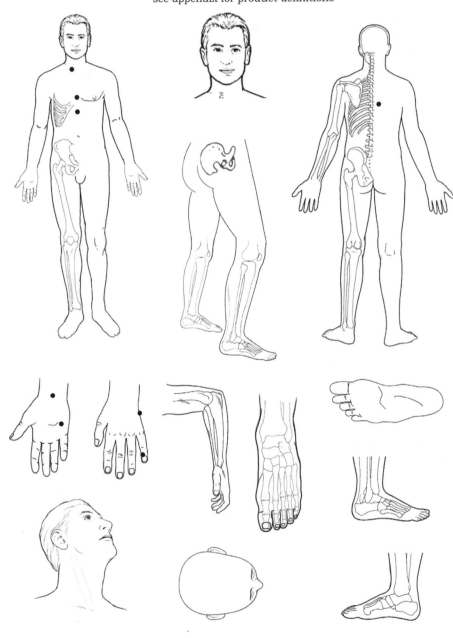

44

Arterial Insufficiency

Emergency Nutritional Daily Menu	Maintenance Nutritional Daily Menu
Glyco: 6 tsp Phyto: 2 tsp Pre-Hormone: 6 tabs Cata-Blend: 6 tabs	Glyco: 2 tsp Phyto: 1 tsp Pre-Hormone: 3 tabs Cata-Blend: 6 tabs

see appendix for product definitions

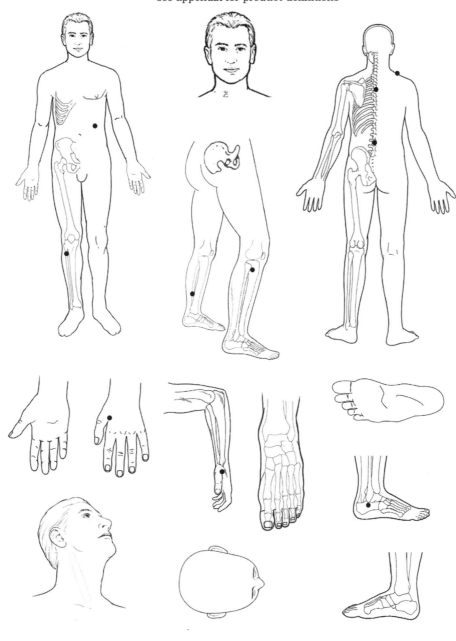

45

Arthralgia

Emergency Nutritional Daily Menu	Maintenance Nutritional Daily Menu
Glyco: 6 tsp Phyto: 2 tsp Pre-Hormone: 6 tabs Cata-Blend: 6 tabs	Glyco: 2 tsp Phyto: 1/2 tsp Pre-Hormone: 4 tabs Cata-Blend: 6 tabs

see appendix for product definitions

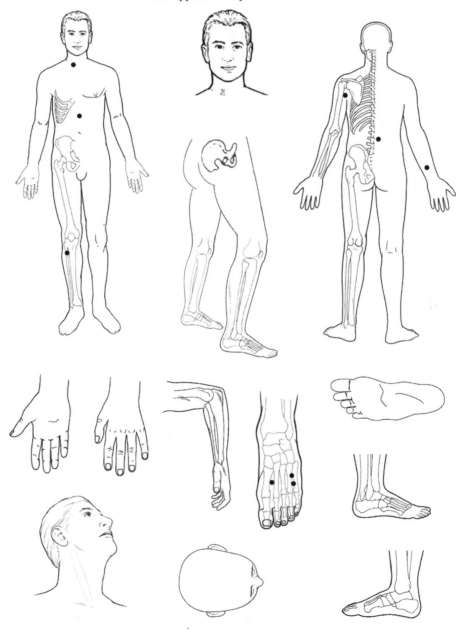

46

Arthritis

Emergency Nutritional Daily Menu	Maintenance Nutritional Daily Menu
Glyco: 6 tsp Phyto: 2 tsp Pre-Hormone: 6 tabs Cata-Blend: 6 tabs	Glyco: 2 tsp Phyto: 1 tsp Pre-Hormone: 4 tabs Cata-Blend: 6 tabs

see appendix for product definitions

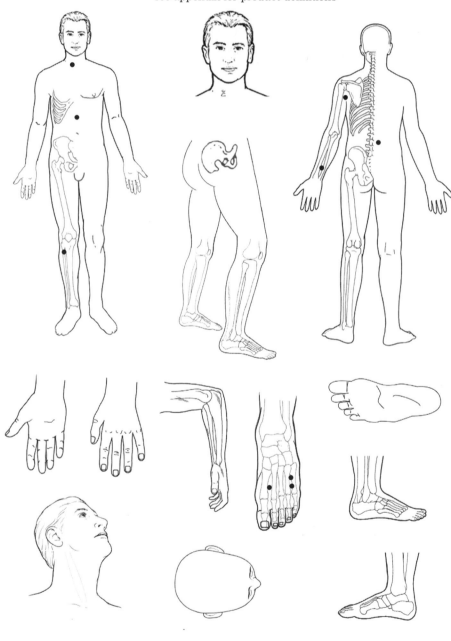

47

AS (Ankylosing Spondylitis)

Emergency Nutritional Daily Menu	Maintenance Nutritional Daily Menu
Glyco: 2 tsp Phyto: 1/2 tsp Pre-Hormone: 6 tabs Cata-Blend: 4 tabs	Glyco: 2 tsp Phyto: 1/2 tsp Pre-Hormone: 3 tabs Cata-Blend: 4 tabs

see appendix for product definitions

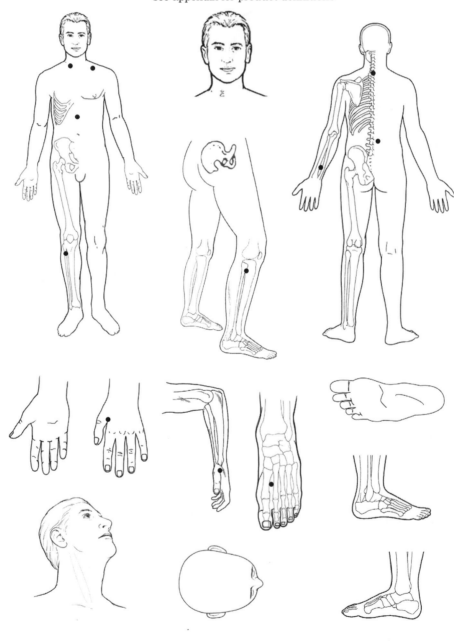

48

ASHD/CAD (Atherosclerotic Heart Disease)

Emergency Nutritional Daily Menu	Maintenance Nutritional Daily Menu
Glyco: 6 tsp Phyto: 3 tsp Pre-Hormone: 4 tabs Cata-Blend: 4 tabs	Glyco: 2 tsp Phyto: 1 tsp Pre-Hormone: 4 tabs Cata-Blend: 4 tabs

see appendix for product definitions

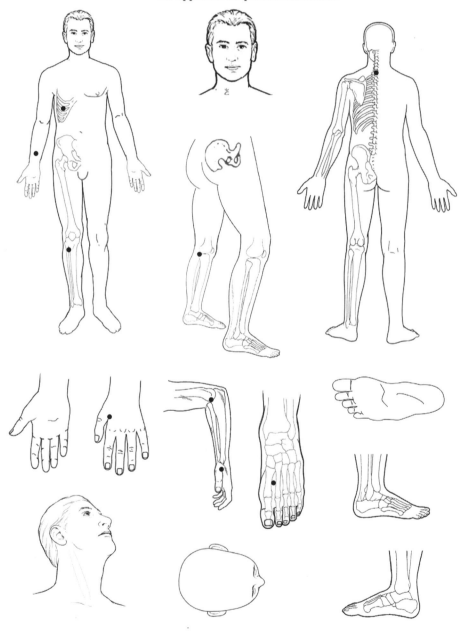

Asthma w/o Status Asthmaticus

Emergency Nutritional Daily Menu	Maintenance Nutritional Daily Menu
Glyco: 6 tsp Phyto: 2 tsp Pre-Hormone: 4 tabs Cata-Blend: 4 tabs	Glyco: 2 tsp Phyto: 1 tsp Pre-Hormone: 3 tabs Cata-Blend: 4 tabs

see appendix for product definitions

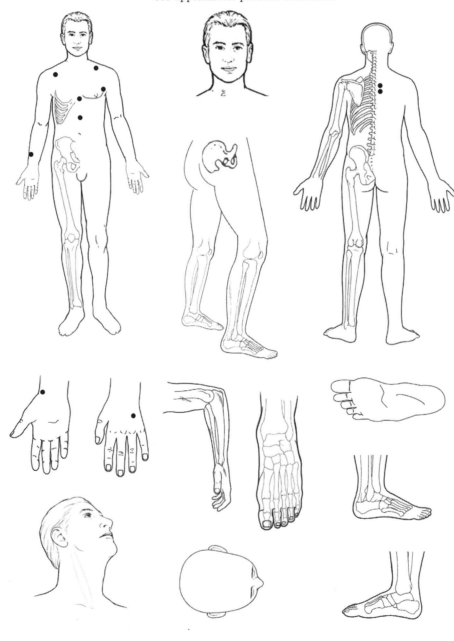

Athlete's Foot

Emergency Nutritional Daily Menu	Maintenance Nutritional Daily Menu
Glyco: 2 tsp Phyto: 1/2 tsp Pre-Hormone: 3 tabs Essentials: 4 tabs	Glyco: 1 tsp Phyto: 1/2 tsp Pre-Hormone: 3 tabs Essentials: 4 tabs

see appendix for product definitions

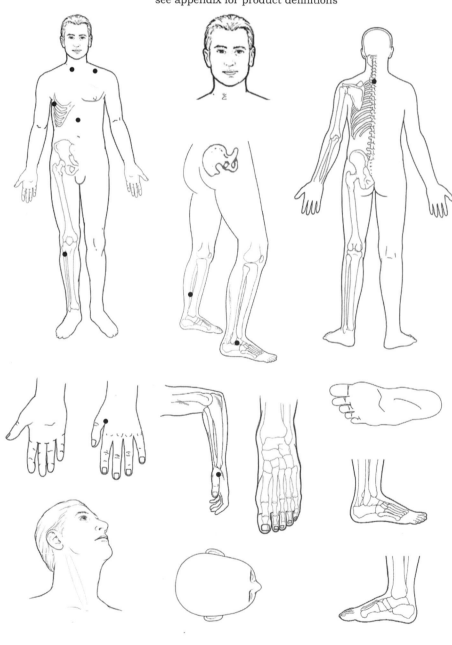

Atrial Fibrillation

Emergency Nutritional Daily Menu	Maintenance Nutritional Daily Menu
Glyco: 6 tsp Phyto: 2 tsp Pre-Hormone: 3 tabs Cata-Blend: 6 tabs	Glyco: 2 tsp Phyto: 1 tsp Pre-Hormone: 3 tabs Cata-Blend: 6 tabs

see appendix for product definitions

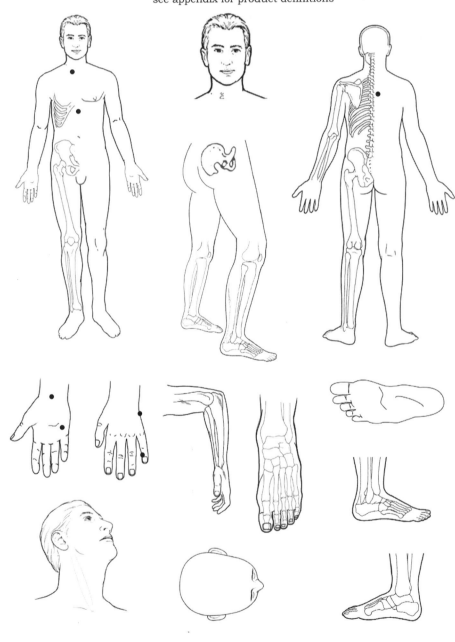

Atrial Flutter

Emergency Nutritional Daily Menu	Maintenance Nutritional Daily Menu
Glyco: 6 tsp Phyto: 2 tsp Pre-Hormone: 3 tabs Cata-Blend: 6 tabs	Glyco: 2 tsp Phyto: 1 tsp Pre-Hormone: 3 tabs Cata-Blend: 6 tabs

see appendix for product definitions

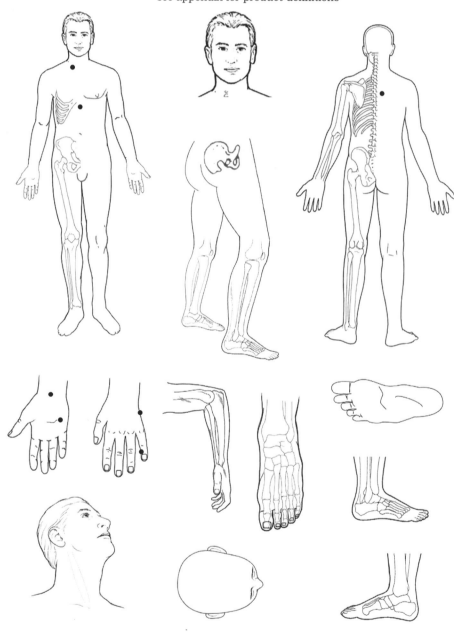

53

Attention Deficit Disorder (ADD)

Emergency Nutritional Daily Menu	Maintenance Nutritional Daily Menu
Glyco: 3 tsp Phyto: 1 tsp Pre-Hormone: 4 tabs Cata-Blend: 4 tabs	Glyco: 2 tsp Phyto: 1 tsp Pre-Hormone: 3 tabs Cata-Blend: 4 tabs

see appendix for product definitions

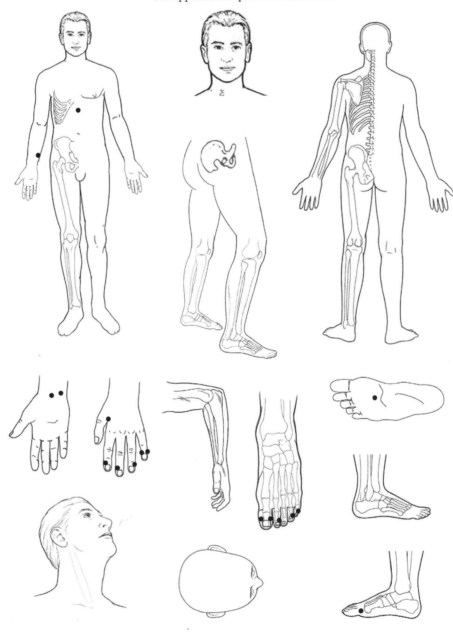

Autism

Emergency Nutritional Daily Menu	Maintenance Nutritional Daily Menu
Glyco: 6 tsp Phyto: 2 tsp Pre-Hormone: 6 tabs Cata-Blend: 4 tabs	Glyco: 2 tsp Phyto: 1 tsp Pre-Hormone: 3 tabs Cata-Blend: 4 tabs

see appendix for product definitions

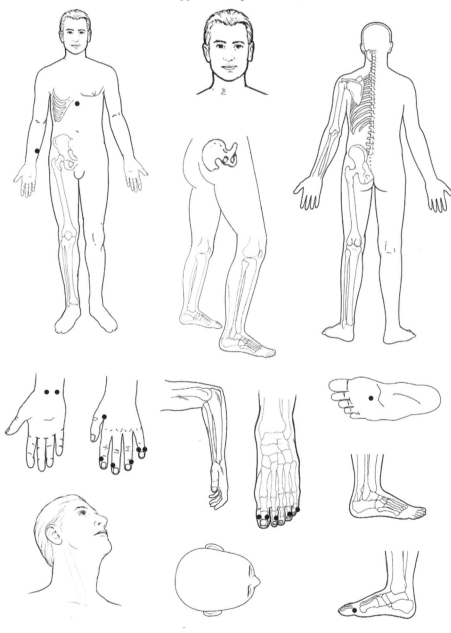

Back Pain w/ Radiation

Emergency Nutritional Daily Menu	Maintenance Nutritional Daily Menu
Glyco: 6 tsp Phyto: 2 tsp Pre-Hormone: 6 tabs Cata-Blend: 4 tabs	Glyco: 2 tsp Phyto: 1 tsp Pre-Hormone: 3 tabs Cata-Blend: 4 tabs

see appendix for product definitions

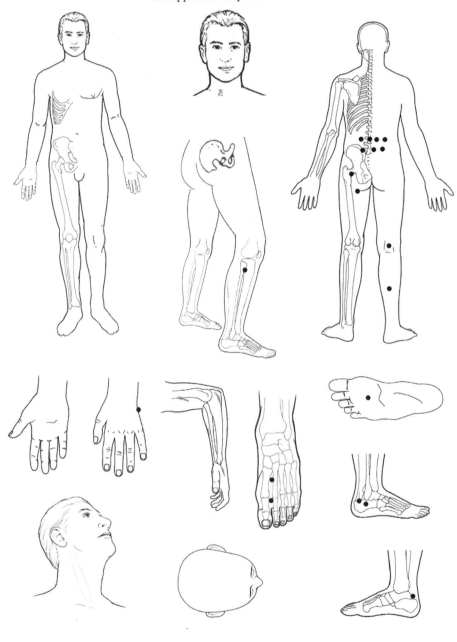

56

Bacteremia (Not Septicemia)

Emergency Nutritional Daily Menu	Maintenance Nutritional Daily Menu
Glyco: 6 tsp Phyto: 1 tsp Pre-Hormone: 6 tabs Cata-Blend: 4 tabs	Glyco: 1 tsp Phyto: 1/2 tsp Pre-Hormone: 3 tabs Cata-Blend: 4 tabs

see appendix for product definitions

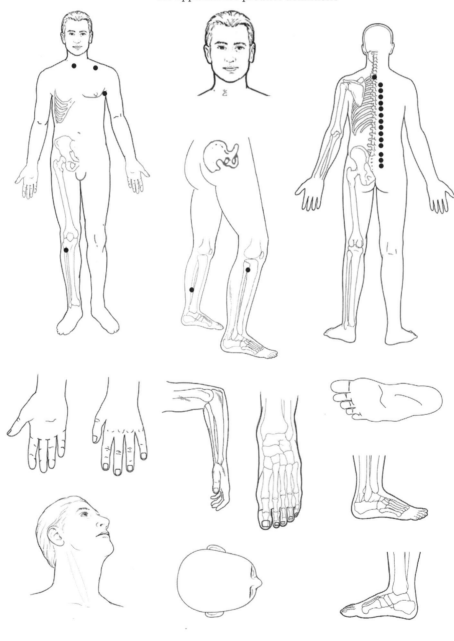

Bacterial Infection

Emergency Nutritional Daily Menu	Maintenance Nutritional Daily Menu
Glyco: 6 tsp Phyto: 2 tsp Pre-Hormone: 6 tabs Essentials: 6 tabs	Glyco: 1 tsp Phyto: 1/2 tsp Pre-Hormone: 3 tabs Essentials: 4 tabs

see appendix for product definitions

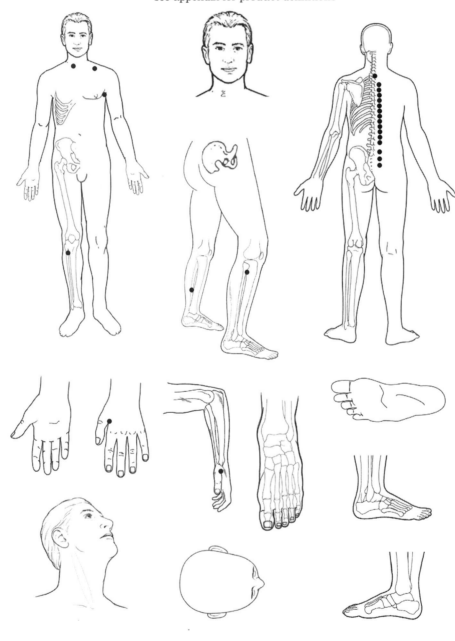

58

Bed Sores

Emergency Nutritional Daily Menu	Maintenance Nutritional Daily Menu
Glyco: 6 tsp Phyto: 1 tsp Pre-Hormone: 4 tabs Cata-Blend: 6 tabs	Glyco: 2 tsp Phyto: 1 tsp Pre-Hormone: 3 tabs Cata-Blend: 4 tabs

see appendix for product definitions

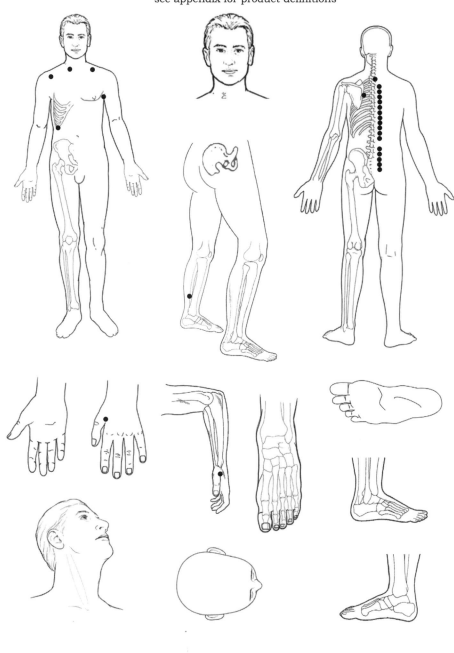

59

Bell's Palsy

Emergency Nutritional Daily Menu	Maintenance Nutritional Daily Menu
Glyco: 3 tsp Phyto: 1/2 tsp Pre-Hormone: 4 tabs Cata-Blend: 4 tabs	Glyco: 2 tsp Phyto: 1/2 tsp Pre-Hormone: 3 tabs Cata-Blend: 4 tabs

see appendix for product definitions

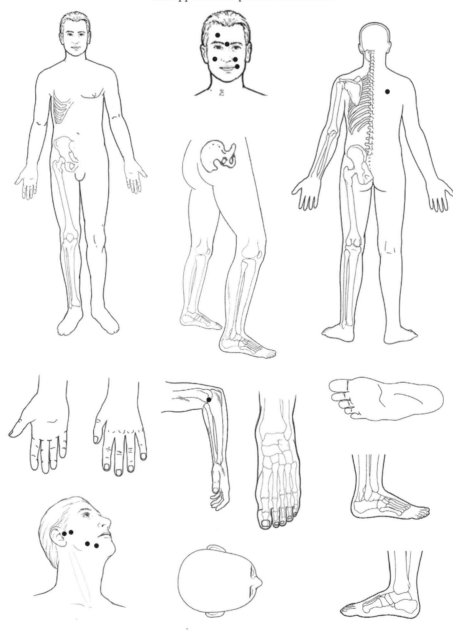

Bipolar Affective Disorder

Emergency Nutritional Daily Menu	Maintenance Nutritional Daily Menu
Glyco: 6 tsp Phyto: 1 tsp Pre-Hormone: 6 tabs Cata-Blend: 6 tabs	Glyco: 2 tsp Phyto: 1 tsp Pre-Hormone: 4 tabs Cata-Blend: 4 tabs

see appendix for product definitions

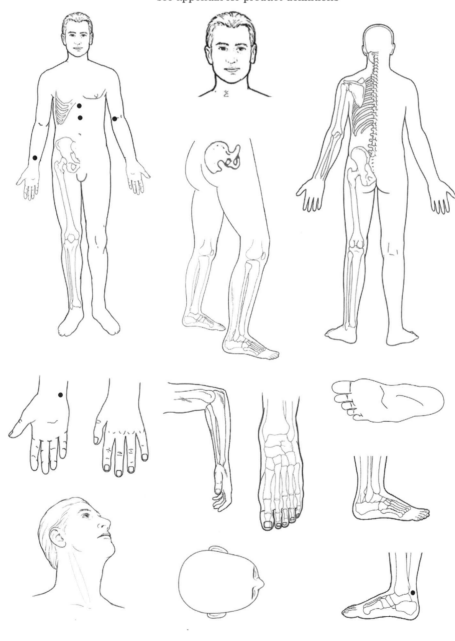

Bladder Problems

Emergency Nutritional Daily Menu	Maintenance Nutritional Daily Menu
Glyco: 3 tsp Phyto: 1/2 tsp Pre-Hormone: 3 tabs Essentials: 4 tabs	Glyco: 1 tsp Phyto: 1/2 tsp Pre-Hormone: 3 tabs Essentials: 4 tabs

see appendix for product definitions

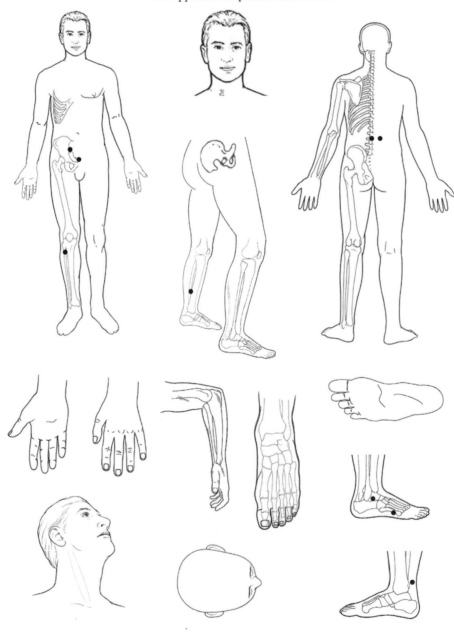

Bloating / Flatulence / Gas

Emergency Nutritional Daily Menu	Maintenance Nutritional Daily Menu
Glyco: 3 tsp Phyto: 1/2 tsp Pre-Hormone: 4 tabs Essentials: 4 tabs	Glyco: 1 tsp Phyto: 1/2 tsp Pre-Hormone: 3 tabs Essentials: 4 tabs

see appendix for product definitions

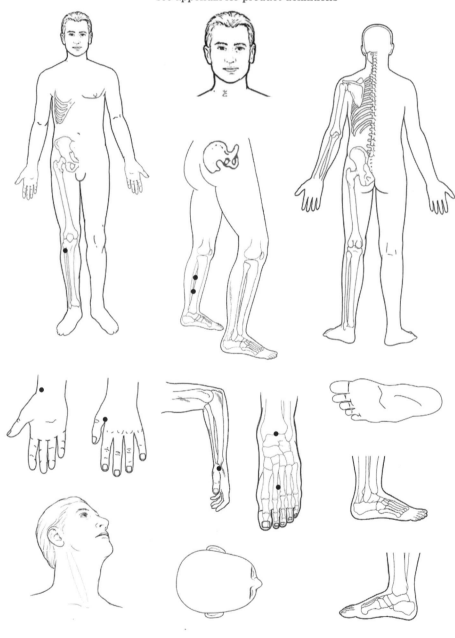

Blocked Tear Duct Lacrimal Duct Obstruction

Emergency Nutritional Daily Menu	Maintenance Nutritional Daily Menu
Glyco: 1 tsp Phyto: 1/2 tsp Pre-Hormone: 3 tabs Essentials: 4 tabs	Glyco: 1/2 tsp Phyto: 1/2 tsp Pre-Hormone: 3 tabs Essentials: 4 tabs

see appendix for product definitions

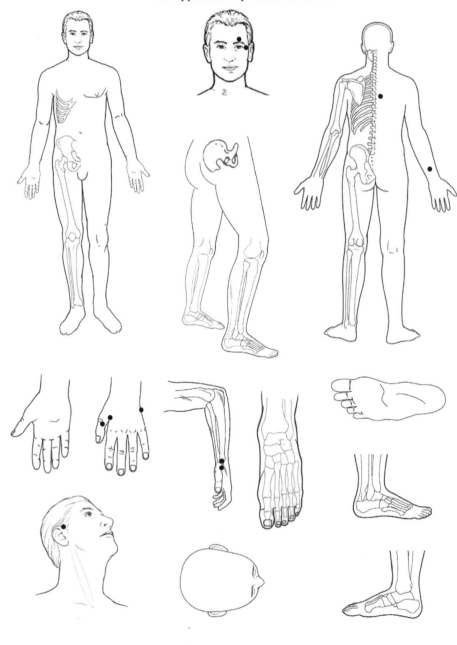

Blood Pressure (Elevated w/o Hypertension)

Emergency Nutritional Daily Menu	Maintenance Nutritional Daily Menu
Glyco: 6 tsp Phyto: 2 tsp Pre-Hormone: 6 tabs Cata-Blend: 4 tabs	Glyco: 2 tsp Phyto: 1 tsp Pre-Hormone: 3 tabs Cata-Blend: 4 tabs

see appendix for product definitions

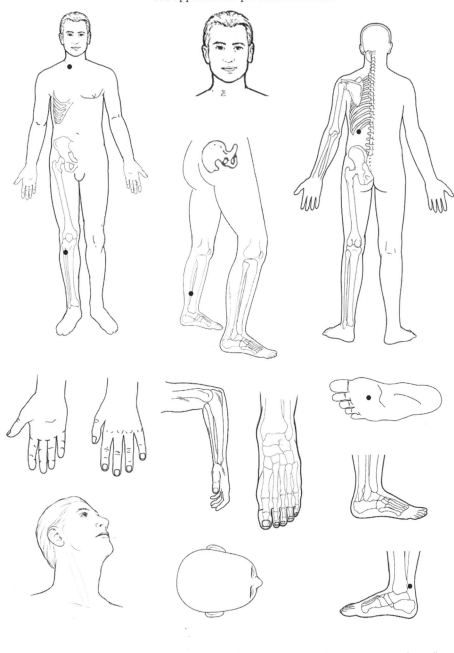

Blood Sugar (Low)

Emergency Nutritional Daily Menu	Maintenance Nutritional Daily Menu
Glyco: 3 tsp Phyto: 2 tsp Pre-Hormone: 6 tabs Essentials: 6 tabs	Glyco: 1 tsp Phyto: 1 tsp Pre-Hormone: 3 tabs Essentials: 4 tabs

see appendix for product definitions

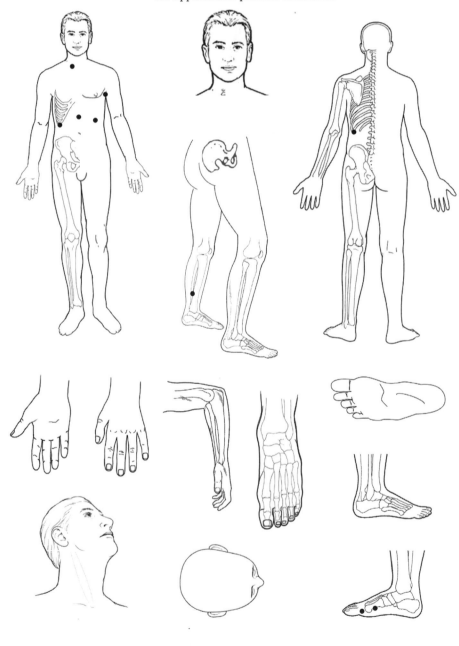

Bowel Detoxification

Emergency Nutritional Daily Menu	Maintenance Nutritional Daily Menu
Glyco: 9 tsp Phyto: 1 tsp Pre-Hormone: 4 tabs Essentials: 4 tabs	Glyco: 1 tsp Phyto: 1 tsp Pre-Hormone: 3 tabs Essentials: 4 tabs

see appendix for product definitions

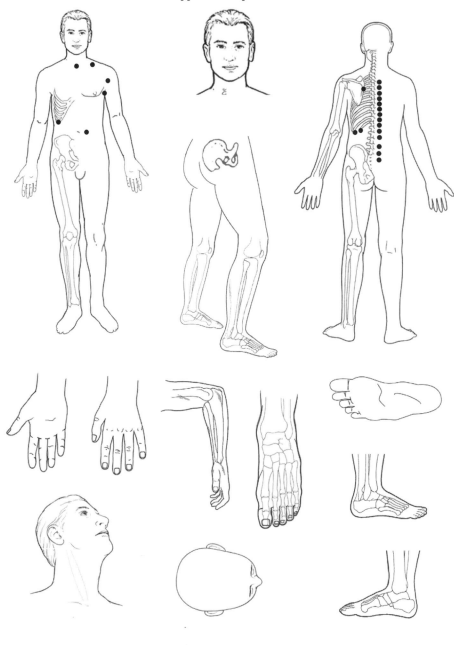

Breast Cyst

Emergency Nutritional Daily Menu	Maintenance Nutritional Daily Menu
Glyco: 3 tsp Phyto: 1 tsp Pre-Hormone: 4 tabs Essentials: 4 tabs	Glyco: 1 tsp Phyto: 1 tsp Pre-Hormone: 4 tabs Essentials: 4 tabs

see appendix for product definitions

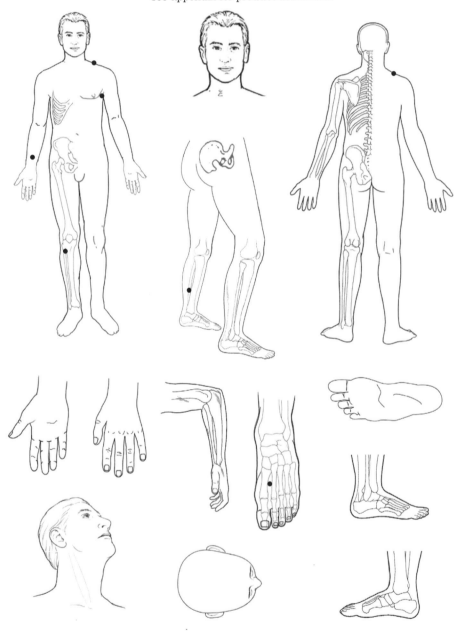

Breast Implants (Leaking)

Emergency Nutritional Daily Menu	Maintenance Nutritional Daily Menu
Glyco: 6 tsp Phyto: 2 tsp Pre-Hormone: 4 tabs Cata-Blend: 6 tabs	Glyco: 2 tsp Phyto: 1 tsp Pre-Hormone: 4 tabs Cata-Blend: 4 tabs

see appendix for product definitions

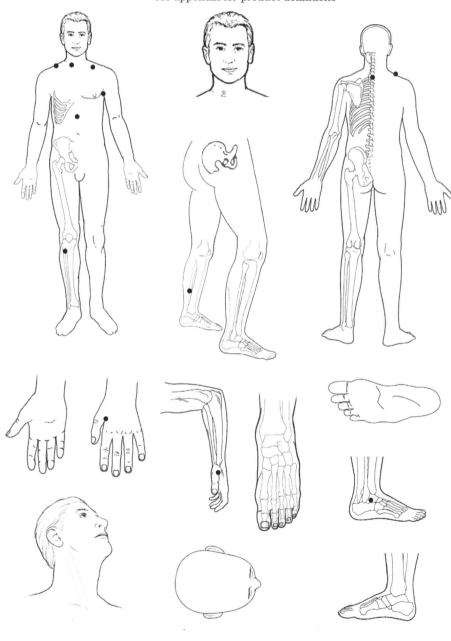

Bronchiectasis

Emergency Nutritional Daily Menu	Maintenance Nutritional Daily Menu
Glyco: 3 tsp Phyto: 2 tsp Pre-Hormone: 4 tabs Cata-Blend: 4 tabs	Glyco: 2 tsp Phyto: 1 tsp Pre-Hormone: 3 tabs Cata-Blend: 4 tabs

see appendix for product definitions

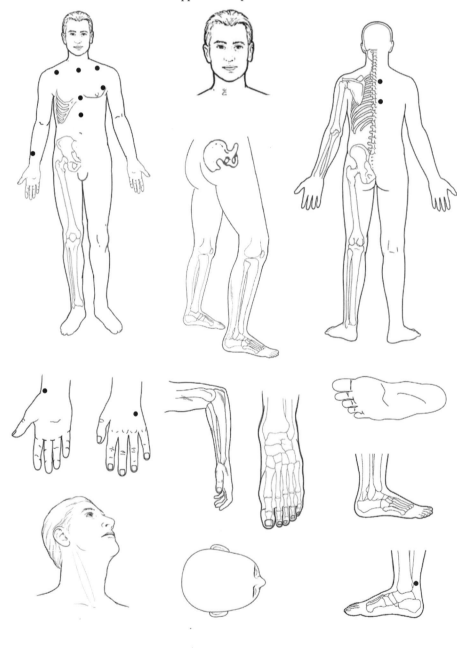

Bronchitis, Chronic

Emergency Nutritional Daily Menu	Maintenance Nutritional Daily Menu
Glyco: 3 tsp Phyto: 1 tsp Pre-Hormone: 4 tabs Cata-Blend: 4 tabs	Glyco: 1 tsp Phyto: 1 tsp Pre-Hormone: 3 tabs Cata-Blend: 4 tabs

see appendix for product definitions

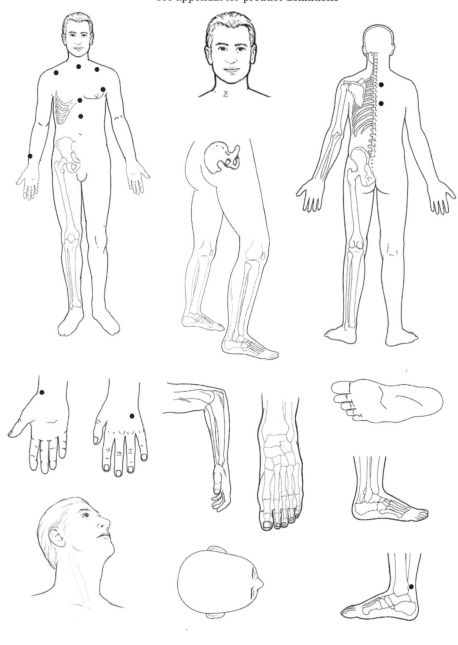

Bruise Easily

Emergency Nutritional Daily Menu	Maintenance Nutritional Daily Menu
Glyco: 3 tsp Phyto: 1 tsp Pre-Hormone: 4 tabs Cata-Blend: 4 tabs	Glyco: 1 tsp Phyto: 1/2 tsp Pre-Hormone: 3 tabs Cata-Blend: 4 tabs

see appendix for product definitions

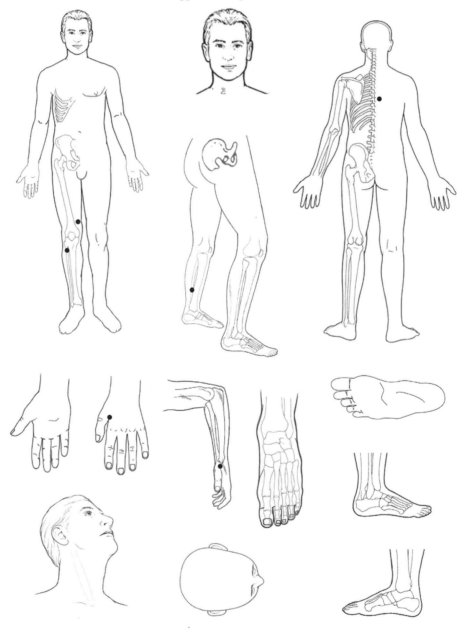

Burns

Emergency Nutritional Daily Menu	Maintenance Nutritional Daily Menu
Glyco: 9 tsp Phyto: 1 tsp Pre-Hormone: 6 tabs Cata-Blend: 6 tabs	Glyco: 1 tsp Phyto: 1 tsp Pre-Hormone: 3 tabs Cata-Blend: 4 tabs

see appendix for product definitions

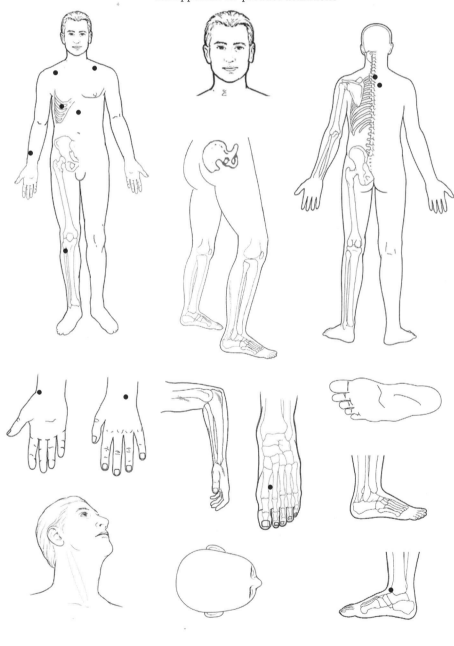

Bursitis

Emergency Nutritional Daily Menu	Maintenance Nutritional Daily Menu
Glyco: 3 tsp Phyto: 1 tsp Pre-Hormone: 6 tabs Cata-Blend: 6 tabs	Glyco: 1 tsp Phyto: 1 tsp Pre-Hormone: 3 tabs Cata-Blend: 4 tabs

see appendix for product definitions

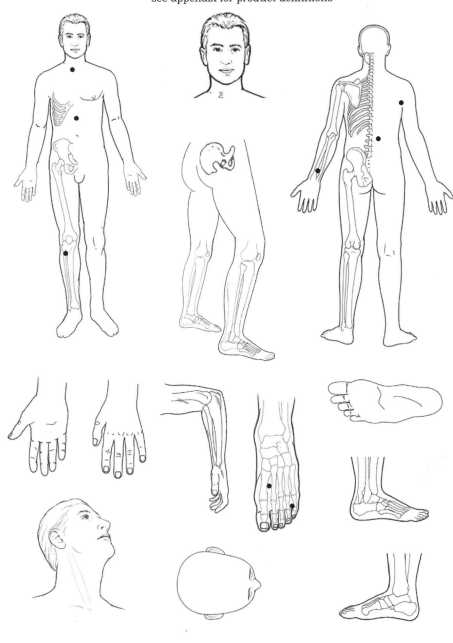

Cancer

Emergency Nutritional Daily Menu	Maintenance Nutritional Daily Menu
Glyco: 12 tsp Phyto: 6 tsp Pre-Hormone: 6 tabs Cata-Blend: 6 tabs	Glyco: 3 tsp Phyto: 3 tsp Pre-Hormone: 4 tabs Cata-Blend: 6 tabs

see appendix for product definitions

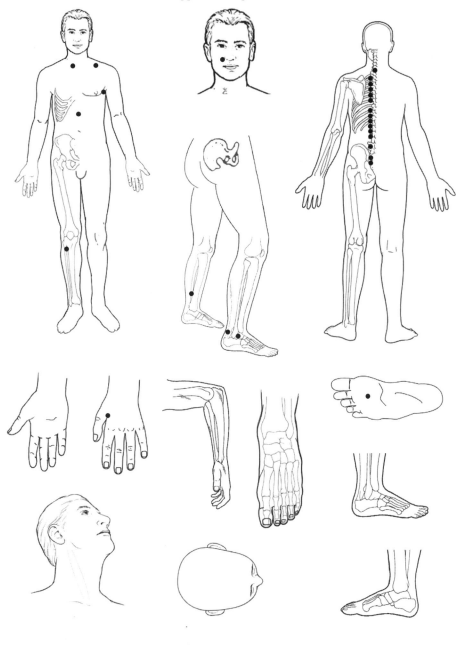

Candidiasis

Emergency Nutritional Daily Menu	Maintenance Nutritional Daily Menu
Glyco: 6 tsp Phyto: 2 tsp Pre-Hormone: 4 tabs Cata-Blend: 4 tabs	Glyco: 2 tsp Phyto: 1 tsp Pre-Hormone: 3 tabs Cata-Blend: 4 tabs

see appendix for product definitions

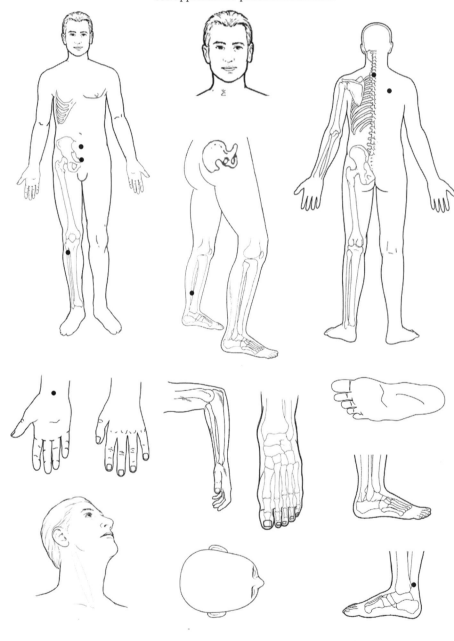

Candidiasis (Oral)

Emergency Nutritional Daily Menu	Maintenance Nutritional Daily Menu
Glyco: 6 tsp Phyto: 2 tsp Pre-Hormone: 4 tabs Cata-Blend: 4 tabs	Glyco: 1 tsp Phyto: 1 tsp Pre-Hormone: 3 tabs Cata-Blend: 4 tabs

see appendix for product definitions

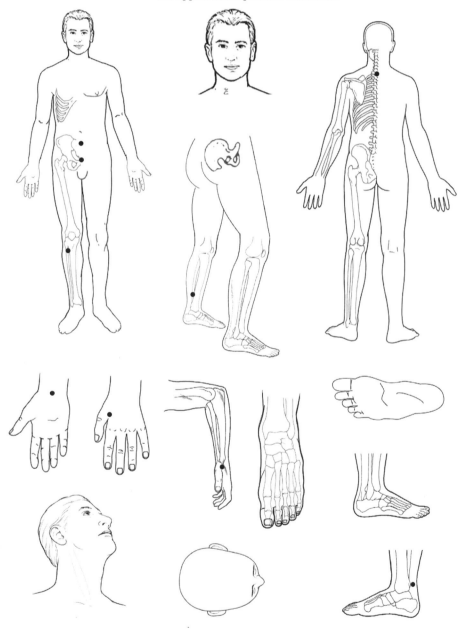

77

Canker Sores

Emergency Nutritional Daily Menu	Maintenance Nutritional Daily Menu
Glyco: 3 tsp Phyto: 1 tsp Pre-Hormone: 3 tabs Essentials: 4 tabs	Glyco: 1 tsp Phyto: 1/2 tsp Pre-Hormone: 3 tabs Essentials: 4 tabs

see appendix for product definitions

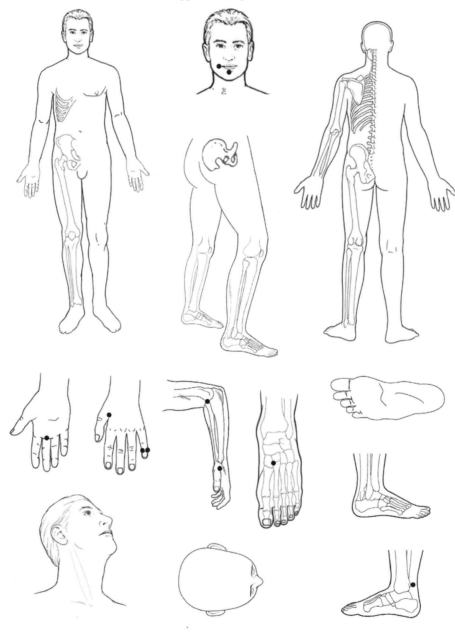

Cardiomyopathy

Emergency Nutritional Daily Menu	Maintenance Nutritional Daily Menu
Glyco: 6 tsp Phyto: 2 tsp Pre-Hormone: 4 tabs Cata-Blend: 6 tabs	Glyco: 2 tsp Phyto: 1 tsp Pre-Hormone: 3 tabs Cata-Blend: 6 tabs

see appendix for product definitions

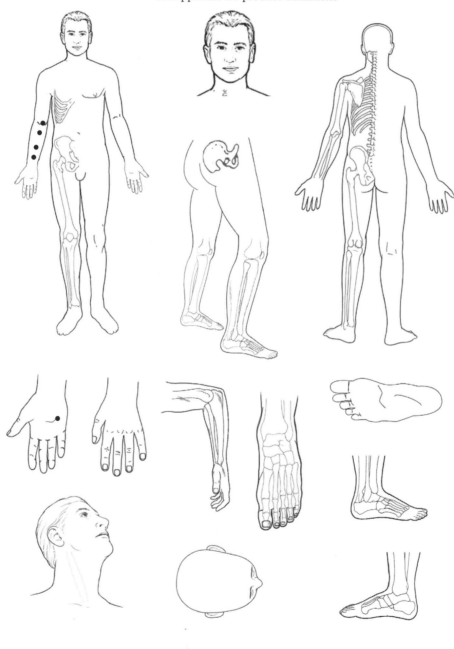

Cellulitis Abscess

Emergency Nutritional Daily Menu	Maintenance Nutritional Daily Menu
Glyco: 6 tsp Phyto: 1 tsp Pre-Hormone: 4 tabs Essentials: 4 tabs	Glyco: 1 tsp Phyto: 1 tsp Pre-Hormone: 3 tabs Essentials: 4 tabs

see appendix for product definitions

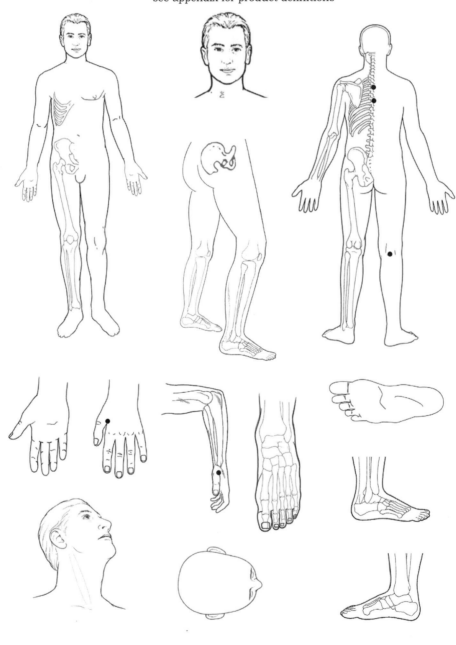

80

Cerebral Aneurysm (Nonruptured)

Emergency Nutritional Daily Menu	Maintenance Nutritional Daily Menu
Glyco: 6 tsp Phyto: 2 tsp Pre-Hormone: 4 tabs Cata-Blend: 4 tabs	Glyco: 2 tsp Phyto: 1 tsp Pre-Hormone: 3 tabs Cata-Blend: 4 tabs

see appendix for product definitions

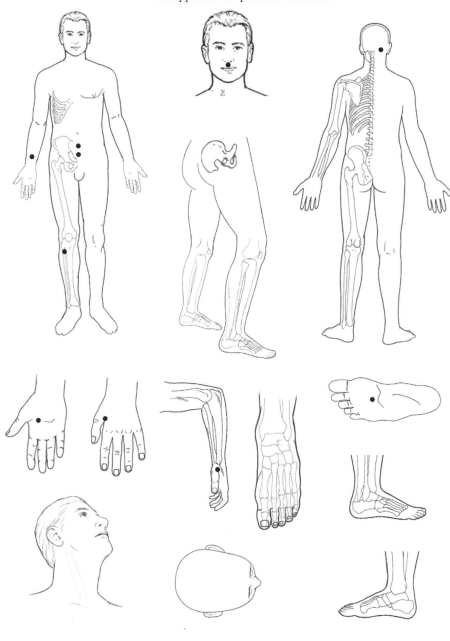

Cerebral Arteriosclerosis

Emergency Nutritional Daily Menu	Maintenance Nutritional Daily Menu
Glyco: 6 tsp Phyto: 2 tsp Pre-Hormone: 4 tabs Cata-Blend: 4 tabs	Glyco: 2 tsp Phyto: 2 tsp Pre-Hormone: 3 tabs Cata-Blend: 4 tabs

see appendix for product definitions

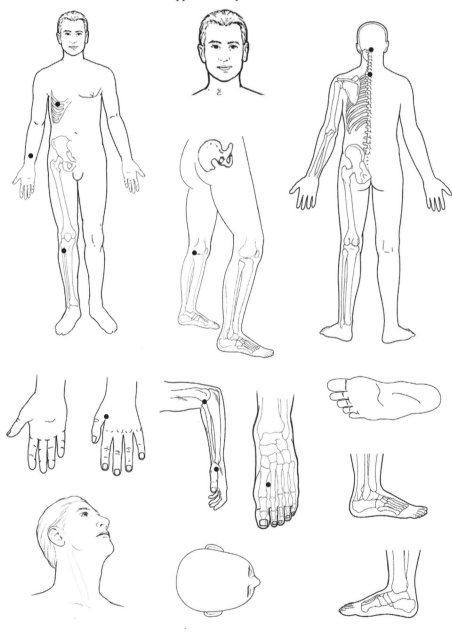

82

Cerebral Hemorrhage (Intracranial)

Emergency Nutritional Daily Menu	Maintenance Nutritional Daily Menu
Glyco: 9 tsp Phyto: 2 tsp Pre-Hormone: 4 tabs Cata-Blend: 6 tabs	Glyco: 2 tsp Phyto: 1 tsp Pre-Hormone: 3 tabs Cata-Blend: 4 tabs

see appendix for product definitions

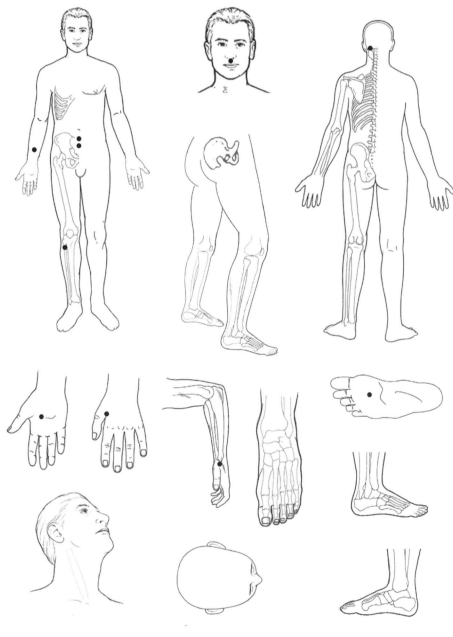

Cerebrovascular Disease

Emergency Nutritional Daily Menu	Maintenance Nutritional Daily Menu
Glyco: 6 tsp Phyto: 2 tsp Pre-Hormone: 4 tabs Cata-Blend: 4 tabs	Glyco: 2 tsp Phyto: 1 tsp Pre-Hormone: 3 tabs Cata-Blend: 4 tabs

see appendix for product definitions

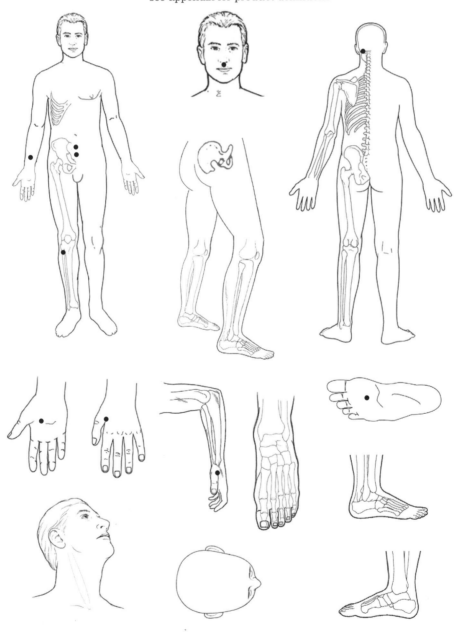

Cervical Dysplasia

Emergency Nutritional Daily Menu	Maintenance Nutritional Daily Menu
Glyco: 6 tsp Phyto: 2 tsp Pre-Hormone: 4 tabs Essentials: 4 tabs	Glyco: 2 tsp Phyto: 1 tsp Pre-Hormone: 3 tabs Essentials: 4 tabs

see appendix for product definitions

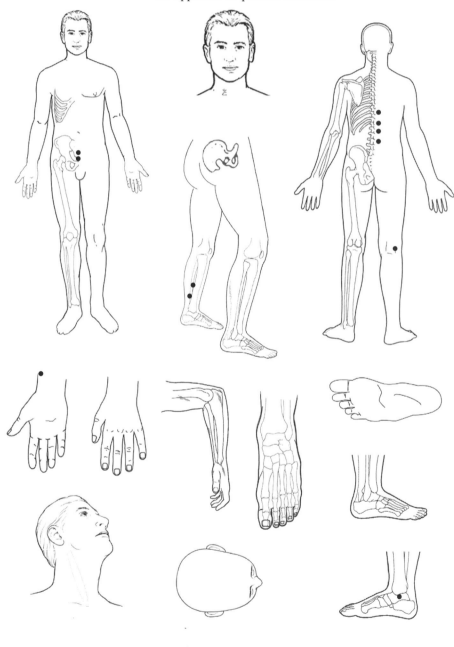

Cervicitis

Emergency Nutritional Daily Menu	Maintenance Nutritional Daily Menu
Glyco: 3 tsp Phyto: 1 tsp Pre-Hormone: 6 tabs Cata-Blend: 4 tabs	Glyco: 2 tsp Phyto: 1/2 tsp Pre-Hormone: 3 tabs Cata-Blend: 4 tabs

see appendix for product definitions

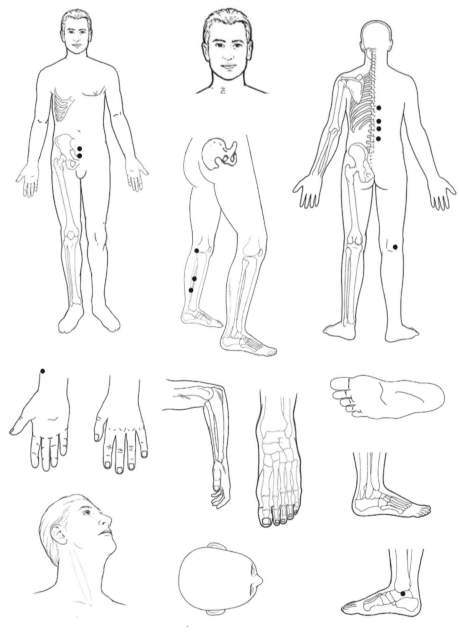

Chest Wall Pain (Costochondritis)

Emergency Nutritional Daily Menu	Maintenance Nutritional Daily Menu
Glyco: 3 tsp Phyto: 1 tsp Pre-Hormone: 6 tabs Essentials: 4 tabs	Glyco: 1 tsp Phyto: 1/2 tsp Pre-Hormone: 3 tabs Essentials: 4 tabs

see appendix for product definitions

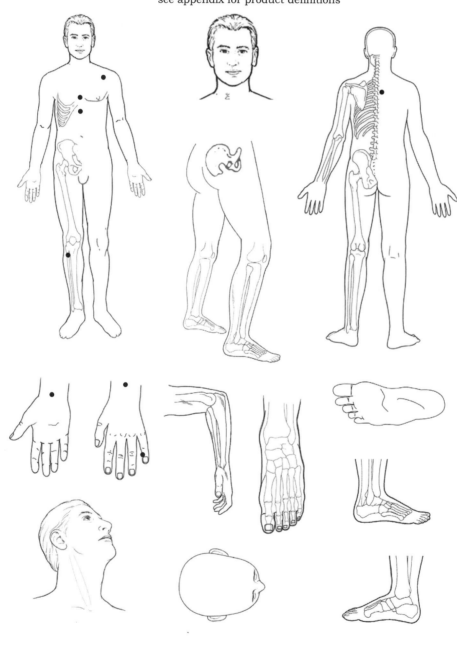

87

Chickenpox

Emergency Nutritional Daily Menu	Maintenance Nutritional Daily Menu
Glyco: 6 tsp Phyto: 1 tsp Pre-Hormone: 4 tabs Essentials: 4 tabs	Glyco: 1 tsp Phyto: 1/2 tsp Pre-Hormone: 3 tabs Essentials: 4 tabs

see appendix for product definitions

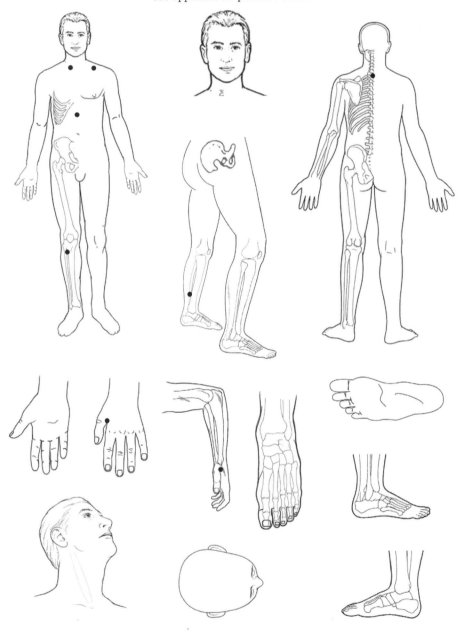

Chlamydia

Emergency Nutritional Daily Menu	Maintenance Nutritional Daily Menu
Glyco: 3 tsp Phyto: 1 tsp Pre-Hormone: 3 tabs Essentials: 6 tabs	Glyco: 1 tsp Phyto: 1/2 tsp Pre-Hormone: 3 tabs Essentials: 4 tabs

see appendix for product definitions

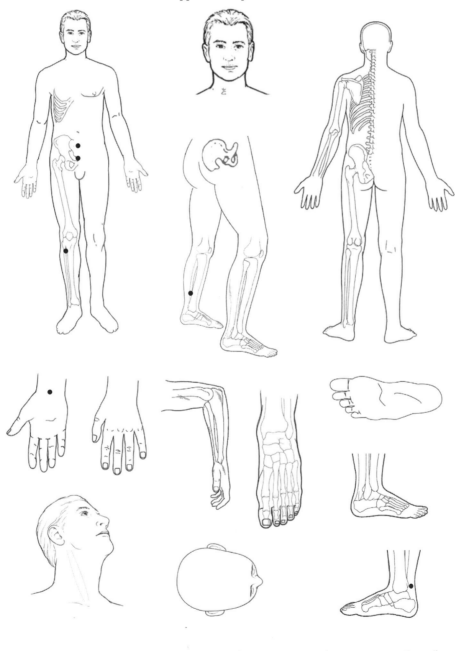

Cholecystitis (Acute)

Emergency Nutritional Daily Menu	Maintenance Nutritional Daily Menu
Glyco: 6 tsp Phyto: 2 tsp Pre-Hormone: 3 tabs Essentials: 6 tabs	Glyco: 3 tsp Phyto: 1 tsp Pre-Hormone: 3 tabs Essentials: 4 tabs

see appendix for product definitions

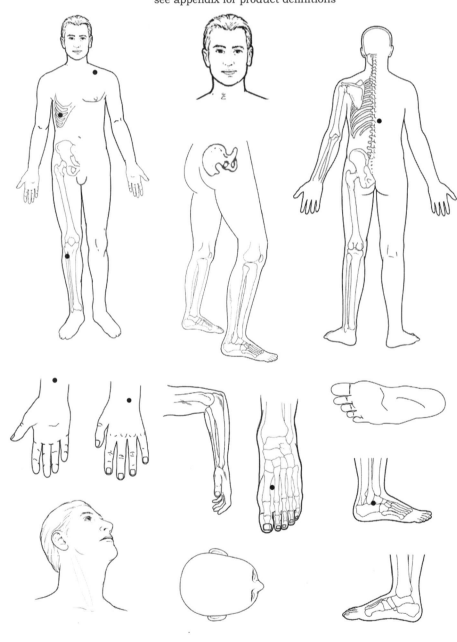

Cholecystitis (Chronic)

Emergency Nutritional Daily Menu	Maintenance Nutritional Daily Menu
Glyco: 3 tsp Phyto: 2 tsp Pre-Hormone: 3 tabs Cata-Blend: 4 tabs	Glyco: 1 tsp Phyto: 1 tsp Pre-Hormone: 3 tabs Cata-Blend: 4 tabs

see appendix for product definitions

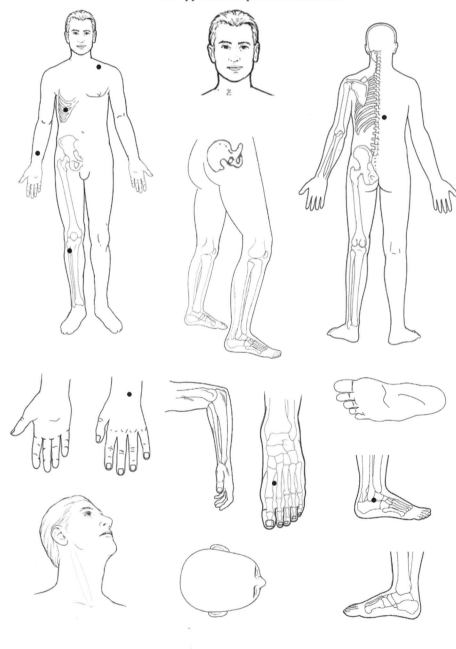

Chronic Fatigue Syndrome

Emergency Nutritional Daily Menu	Maintenance Nutritional Daily Menu
Glyco: 6 tsp Phyto: 2 tsp Pre-Hormone: 6 tabs Cata-Blend: 4 tabs	Glyco: 2 tsp Phyto: 1 tsp Pre-Hormone: 4 tabs Cata-Blend: 4 tabs

see appendix for product definitions

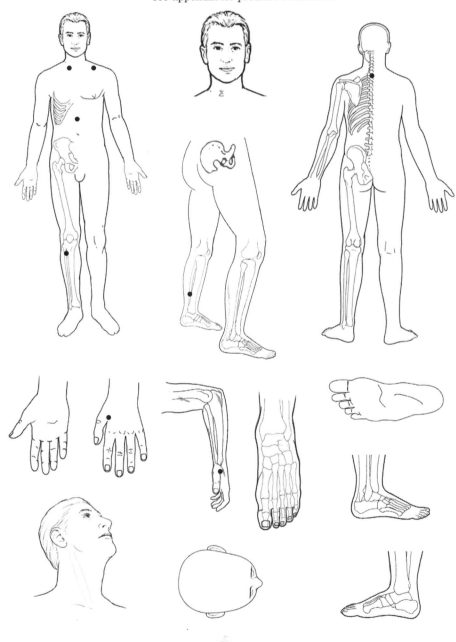

Chronic Ischemic Heart Disease

Emergency Nutritional Daily Menu	Maintenance Nutritional Daily Menu
Glyco: 6 tsp Phyto: 2 tsp Pre-Hormone: 3 tabs Cata-Blend: 4 tabs	Glyco: 3 tsp Phyto: 2 tsp Pre-Hormone: 3 tabs Cata-Blend: 4 tabs

see appendix for product definitions

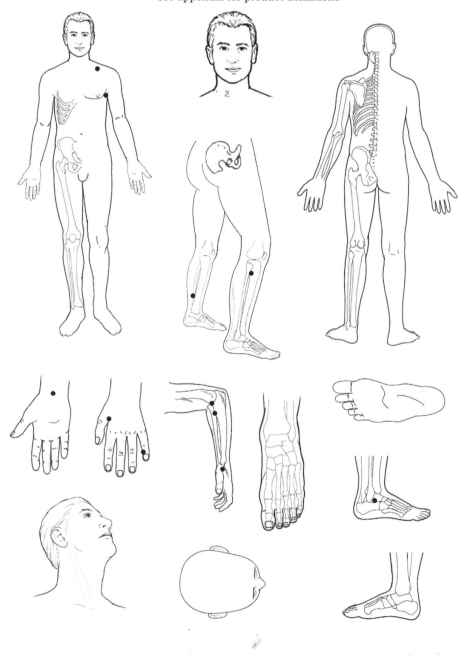

93

Chronic Liver Disease

Emergency Nutritional Daily Menu	Maintenance Nutritional Daily Menu
Glyco: 6 tsp Phyto: 2 tsp Pre-Hormone: 3 tabs Cata-Blend: 4 tabs	Glyco: 2 tsp Phyto: 1 tsp Pre-Hormone: 3 tabs Cata-Blend: 4 tabs

see appendix for product definitions

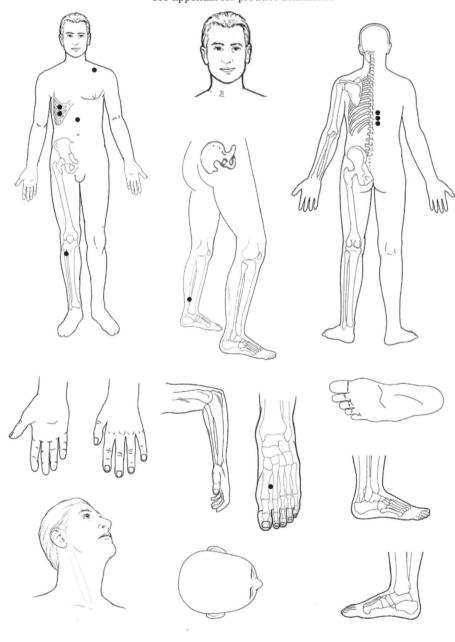

Chronic Skin Ulcer Venous Stasis
(apply soft laser to affect areas)

Emergency Nutritional Daily Menu	Maintenance Nutritional Daily Menu
Glyco: 3 tsp Phyto: 2 tsp Pre-Hormone: 3 tabs Cata-Blend: 4 tabs	Glyco: 2 tsp Phyto: 1 tsp Pre-Hormone: 3 tabs Cata-Blend: 4 tabs

see appendix for product definitions

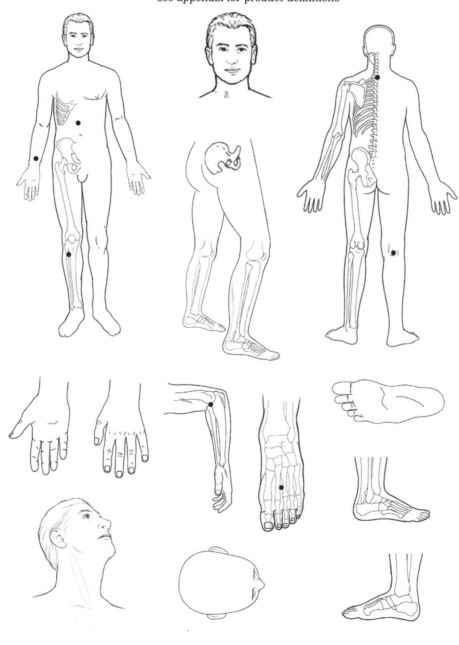

95

Cirrhosis, Alcoholic Liver

Emergency Nutritional Daily Menu	Maintenance Nutritional Daily Menu
Glyco: 6 tsp Phyto: 2 tsp Pre-Hormone: 6 tabs Cata-Blend: 4 tabs	Glyco: 2 tsp Phyto: 1 tsp Pre-Hormone: 3 tabs Cata-Blend: 4 tabs

see appendix for product definitions

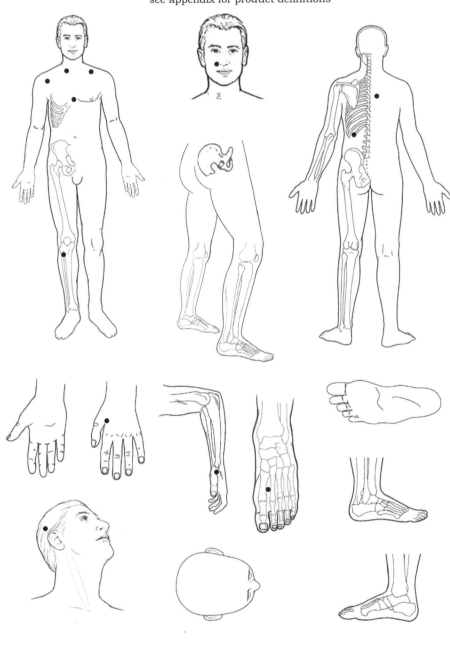

96

Cirrhosis, Nonalcoholic Liver

Emergency Nutritional Daily Menu	Maintenance Nutritional Daily Menu
Glyco: 6 tsp Phyto: 1 tsp Pre-Hormone: 4 tabs Cata-Blend: 4 tabs	Glyco: 2 tsp Phyto: 1 tsp Pre-Hormone: 3 tabs Cata-Blend: 4 tabs

see appendix for product definitions

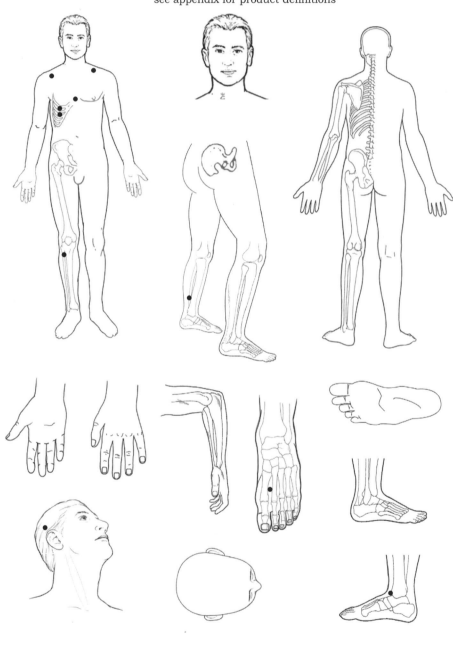

Claudication/Peripheral Vascular Disease

Emergency Nutritional Daily Menu	Maintenance Nutritional Daily Menu
Glyco: 6 tsp Phyto: 2 tsp Pre-Hormone: 6 tabs Cata-Blend: 6 tabs	Glyco: 2 tsp Phyto: 1 tsp Pre-Hormone: 3 tabs Cata-Blend: 4 tabs

see appendix for product definitions

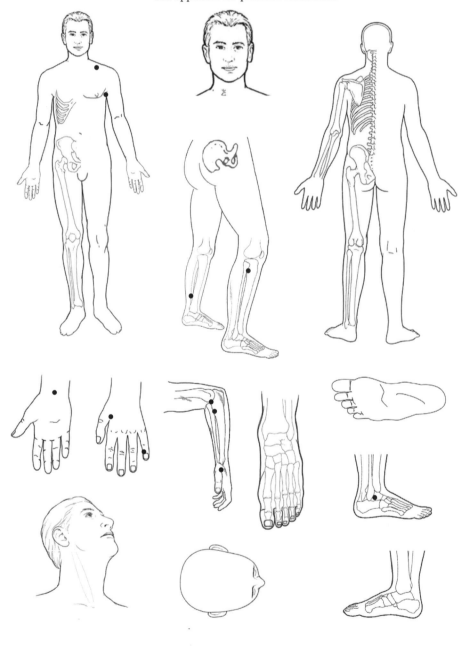

Clostridium Difficile

Emergency Nutritional Daily Menu	Maintenance Nutritional Daily Menu
Glyco: 3 tsp Phyto: 1 tsp Pre-Hormone: 3 tabs Cata-Blend: 6 tabs	Glyco: 1 tsp Phyto: 1/2 tsp Pre-Hormone: 3 tabs Cata-Blend: 4 tabs

see appendix for product definitions

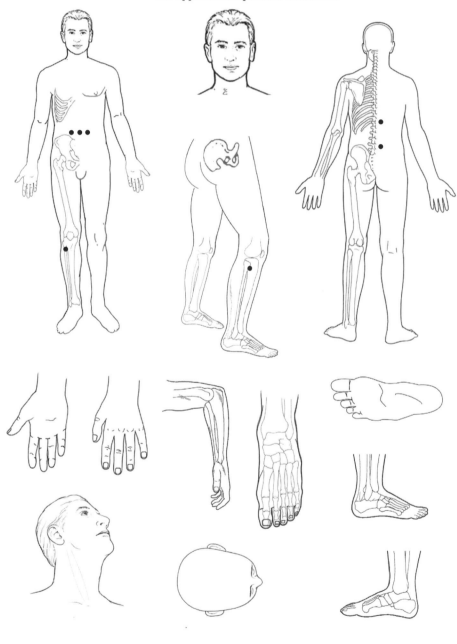

Cold Sores
(apply soft laser to affected areas)

Emergency Nutritional Daily Menu	Maintenance Nutritional Daily Menu
Glyco: 3 tsp Phyto: 1 tsp Pre-Hormone: 3 tabs Essentials: 6 tabs	Glyco: 1 tsp Phyto: 1/2 tsp Pre-Hormone: 3 tabs Essentials: 4 tabs

see appendix for product definitions

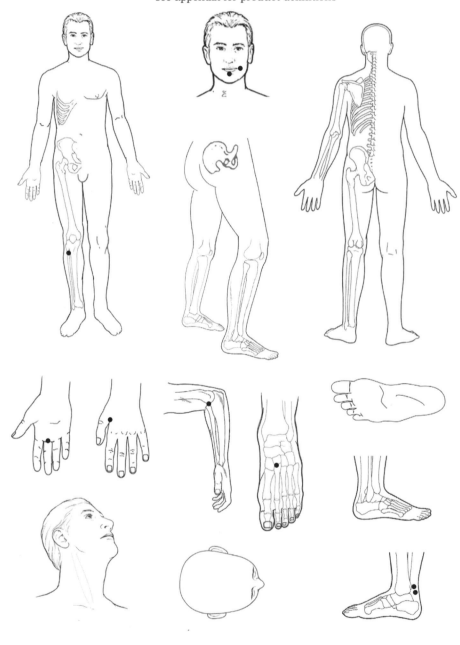

Cold/Flu

Emergency Nutritional Daily Menu	Maintenance Nutritional Daily Menu
Glyco: 3 tsp Phyto: 2 tsp Pre-Hormone: 3 tabs Essentials: 6 tabs	Glyco: 1 tsp Phyto: 1/2 tsp Pre-Hormone: 3 tabs Essentials: 4 tabs

see appendix for product definitions

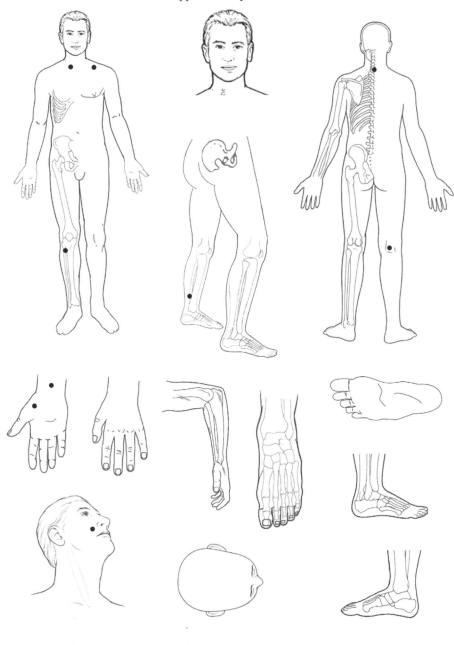

Colitis

Emergency Nutritional Daily Menu	Maintenance Nutritional Daily Menu
Glyco: 6 tsp Phyto: 2 tsp Pre-Hormone: 4 tabs Cata-Blend: 4 tabs	Glyco: 2 tsp Phyto: 1 tsp Pre-Hormone: 3 tabs Cata-Blend: 4 tabs

see appendix for product definitions

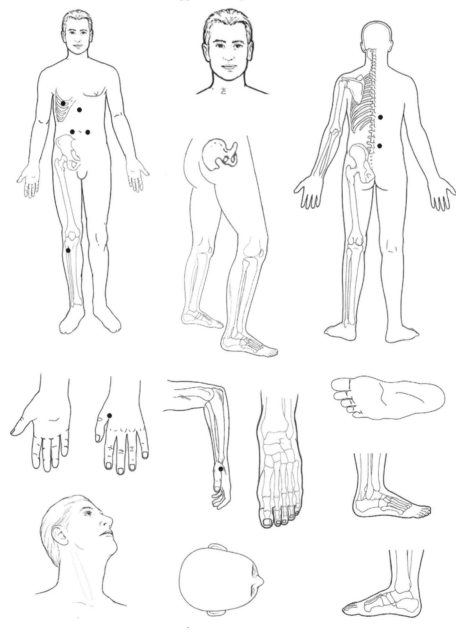

Colon Infection

Emergency Nutritional Daily Menu	Maintenance Nutritional Daily Menu
Glyco: 6 tsp Phyto: 2 tsp Pre-Hormone: 3 tabs Cata-Blend: 4 tabs	Glyco: 1 tsp Phyto: 1 tsp Pre-Hormone: 3 tabs Cata-Blend: 4 tabs

see appendix for product definitions

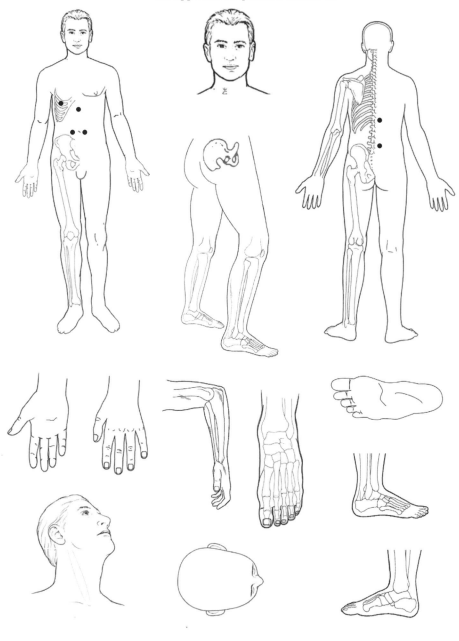

Coma

Emergency Nutritional Daily Menu	Maintenance Nutritional Daily Menu
Glyco: 9 tsp Phyto: 3 tsp Pre-Hormone: 6 tabs Cata-Blend: 6 tabs	Glyco: 3 tsp Phyto: 1 tsp Pre-Hormone: 3 tabs Cata-Blend: 4 tabs

see appendix for product definitions

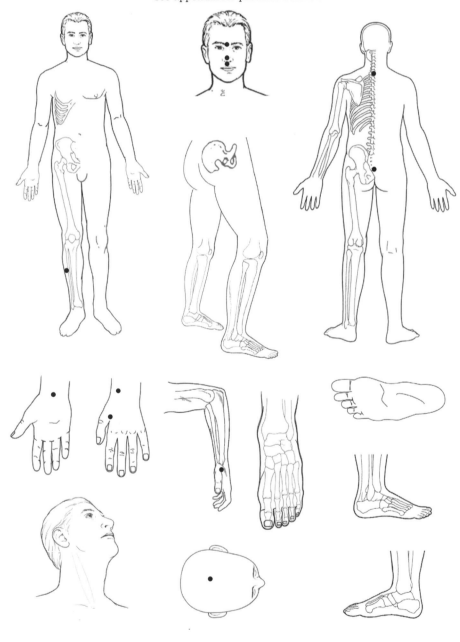

Common Cold

Emergency Nutritional Daily Menu	Maintenance Nutritional Daily Menu
Glyco: 3 tsp Phyto: 2 tsp Pre-Hormone: 3 tabs Essentials: 4 tabs	Glyco: 1/2 tsp Phyto: 1/2 tsp Pre-Hormone: 3 tabs Essentials: 4 tabs

see appendix for product definitions

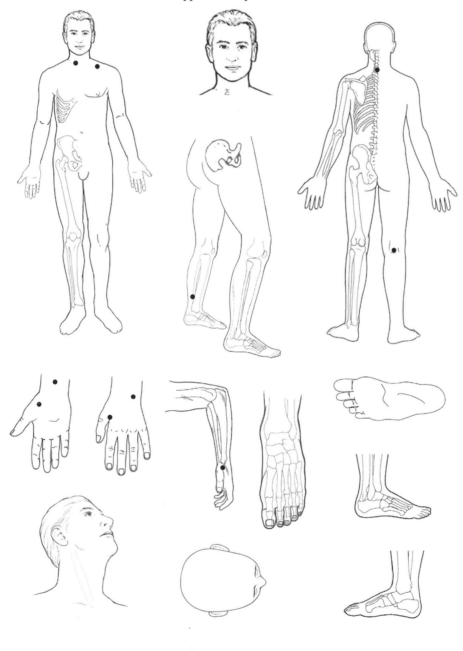

Concussion

Emergency Nutritional Daily Menu	Maintenance Nutritional Daily Menu
Glyco: 9 tsp Phyto: 3 tsp Pre-Hormone: 6 tabs Cata-Blend: 6 tabs	Glyco: 2 tsp Phyto: 1 tsp Pre-Hormone: 3 tabs Cata-Blend: 4 tabs

see appendix for product definitions

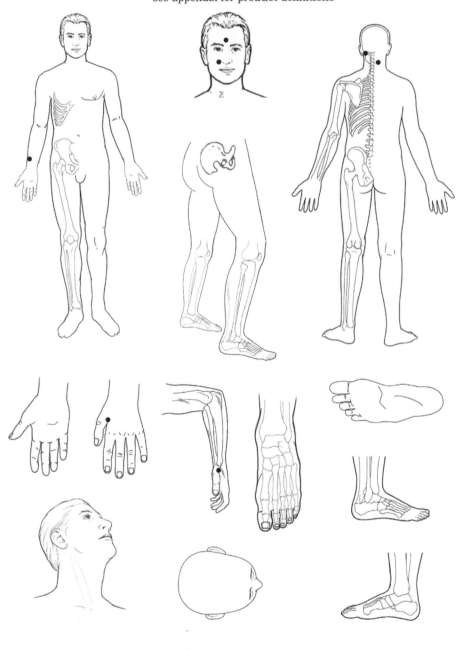

Congenital Heart Defect

Emergency Nutritional Daily Menu	Maintenance Nutritional Daily Menu
Glyco: 6 tsp Phyto: 2 tsp Pre-Hormone: 3 tabs Cata-Blend: 4 tabs	Glyco: 2 tsp Phyto: 1 tsp Pre-Hormone: 3 tabs Cata-Blend: 4 tabs

see appendix for product definitions

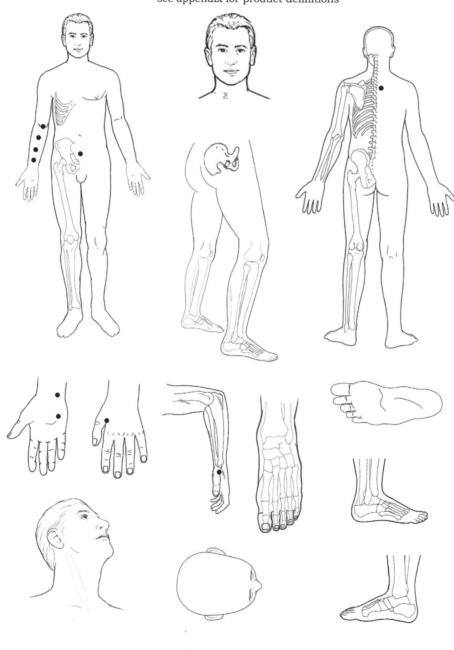

Congestive Heart Failure (CHF)

Emergency Nutritional Daily Menu	Maintenance Nutritional Daily Menu
Glyco: 6 tsp Phyto: 2 tsp Pre-Hormone: 6 tabs Cata-Blend: 4 tabs	Glyco: 2 tsp Phyto: 1 tsp Pre-Hormone: 3 tabs Cata-Blend: 4 tabs

see appendix for product definitions

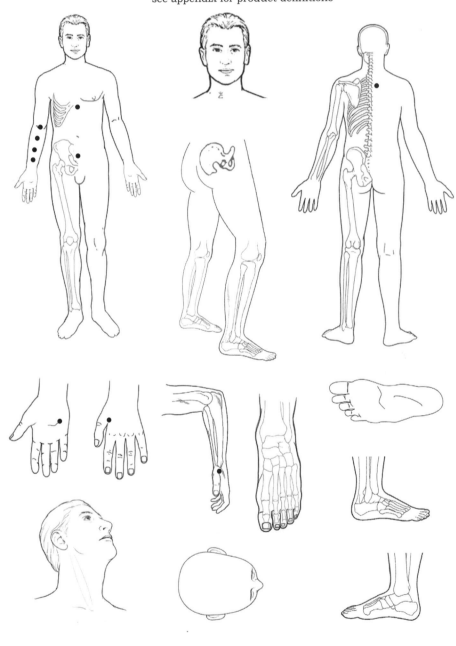

Conjunctivitis

Emergency Nutritional Daily Menu	Maintenance Nutritional Daily Menu
Glyco: 2 tsp Phyto: 1/2 tsp Pre-Hormone: 3 tabs Essentials: 4 tabs	Glyco: 1/2 tsp Phyto: 1/2 tsp Pre-Hormone: 3 tabs Essentials: 4 tabs

see appendix for product definitions

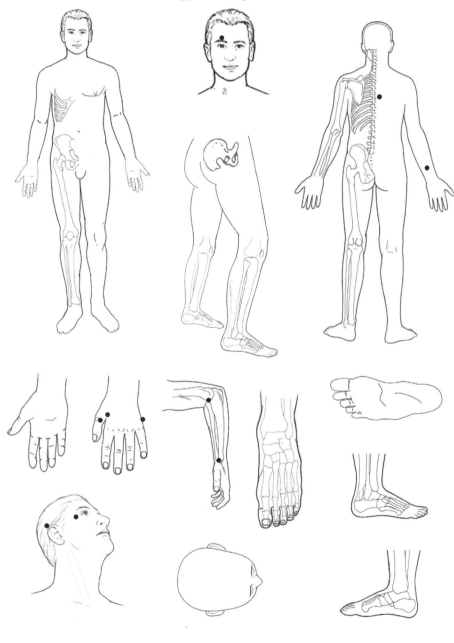

Connective Tissue Disease

Emergency Nutritional Daily Menu	Maintenance Nutritional Daily Menu
Glyco: 9 tsp Phyto: 2 tsp Pre-Hormone: 6 tabs Cata-Blend: 6 tabs	Glyco: 3 tsp Phyto: 1 tsp Pre-Hormone: 3 tabs Cata-Blend: 6 tabs

see appendix for product definitions

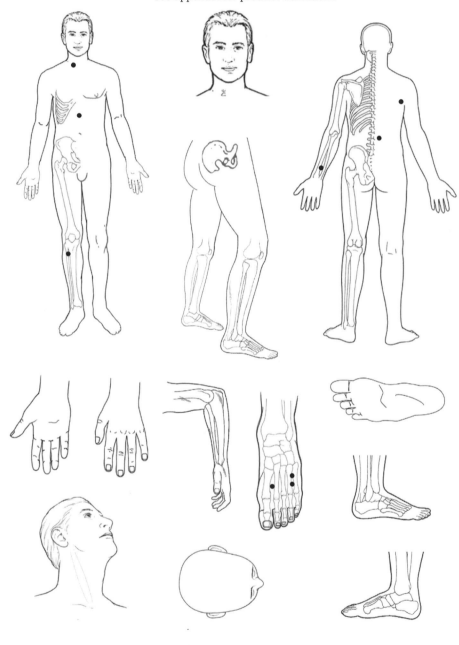

Constipation

Emergency Nutritional Daily Menu	Maintenance Nutritional Daily Menu
Glyco: 3 tsp Phyto: 2 tsp Pre-Hormone: 3 tabs Essentials: 4 tabs	Glyco: 1 tsp Phyto: 1/2 tsp Pre-Hormone: 3 tabs Essentials: 4 tabs

see appendix for product definitions

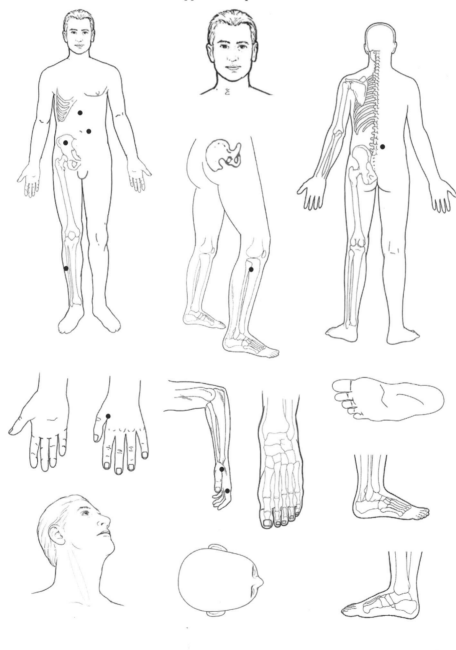

Contact Dermatitis

Emergency Nutritional Daily Menu	Maintenance Nutritional Daily Menu
Glyco: 3 tsp Phyto: 1 tsp Pre-Hormone: 3 tabs Essentials: 4 tabs	Glyco: 1/2 tsp Phyto: 1/2 tsp Pre-Hormone: 3 tabs Essentials: 4 tabs

see appendix for product definitions

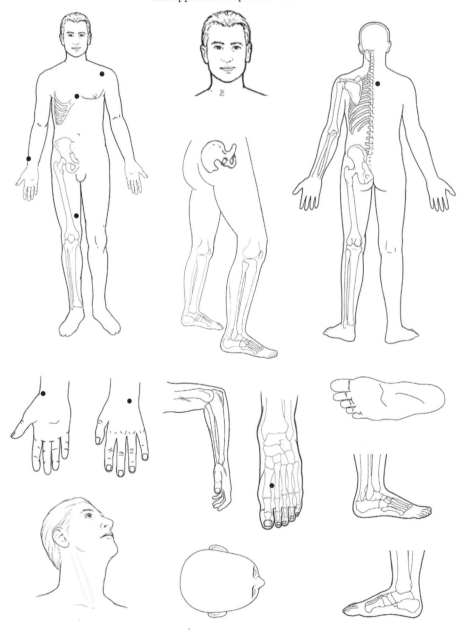

COPD

Emergency Nutritional Daily Menu	Maintenance Nutritional Daily Menu
Glyco: 4 tsp Phyto: 2 tsp Pre-Hormone: 3 tabs Cata-Blend: 4 tabs	Glyco: 2 tsp Phyto: 1 tsp Pre-Hormone: 3 tabs Cata-Blend: 4 tabs

see appendix for product definitions

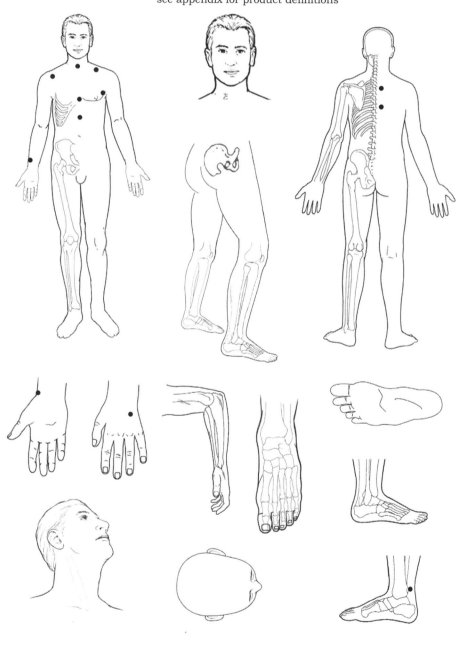

Cor Pulmonale

Emergency Nutritional Daily Menu	Maintenance Nutritional Daily Menu
Glyco: 4 tsp Phyto: 2 tsp Pre-Hormone: 3 tabs Cata-Blend: 4 tabs	Glyco: 2 tsp Phyto: 1 tsp Pre-Hormone: 3 tabs Cata-Blend: 4 tabs

see appendix for product definitions

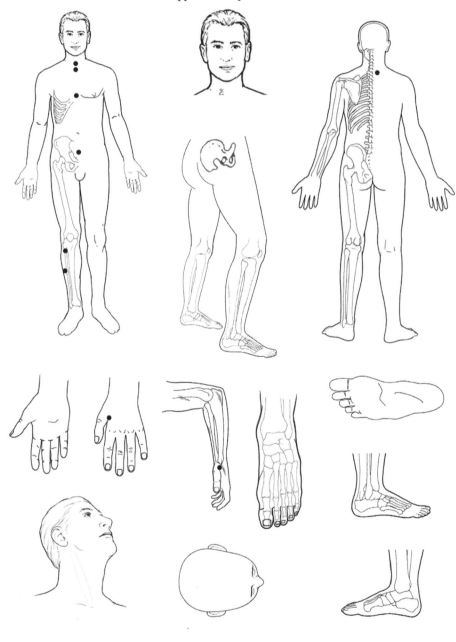

Costochondritis

Emergency Nutritional Daily Menu	Maintenance Nutritional Daily Menu
Glyco: 3 tsp Phyto: 1 tsp Pre-Hormone: 6 tabs Essentials: 4 tabs	Glyco: 1 tsp Phyto: 1/2 tsp Pre-Hormone: 3 tabs Essentials: 4 tabs

see appendix for product definitions

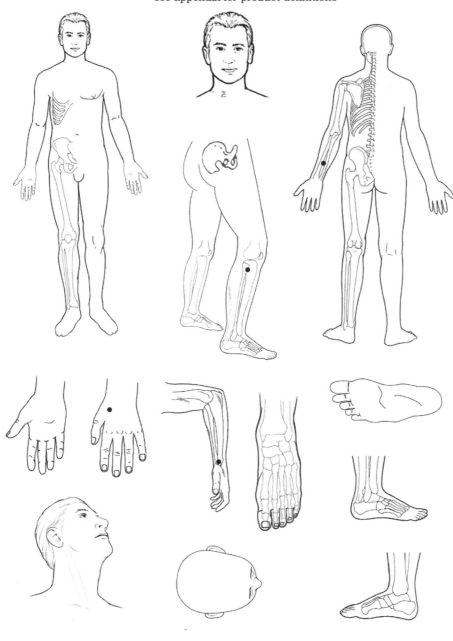

Cough

Emergency Nutritional Daily Menu	Maintenance Nutritional Daily Menu
Glyco: 2 tsp Phyto: 1 tsp Pre-Hormone: 3 tabs Essentials:: 4 tabs	Glyco: 1/2 tsp Phyto: 1/2 tsp Pre-Hormone: 3 tabs Essentials: 4 tabs

see appendix for product definitions

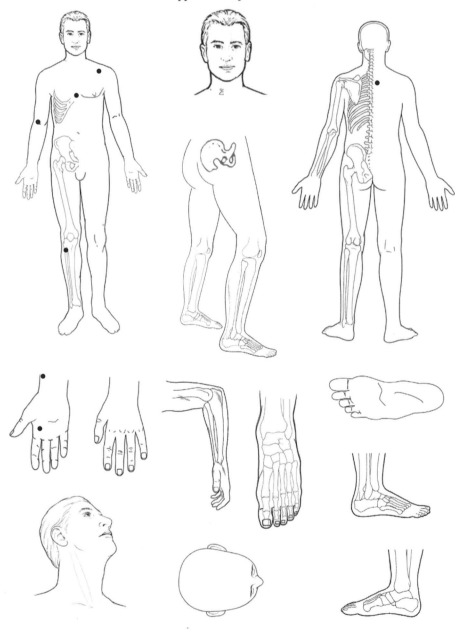

Coumadin Therapy (Long Term)

Emergency Nutritional Daily Menu	Maintenance Nutritional Daily Menu
Glyco: 1 tsp Phyto: 1 tsp Pre-Hormone: 3 tabs Essentials: 4 tabs	Glyco: 1 tsp Phyto: 1/2 tsp Pre-Hormone: 3 tabs Essentials: 4 tabs

see appendix for product definitions

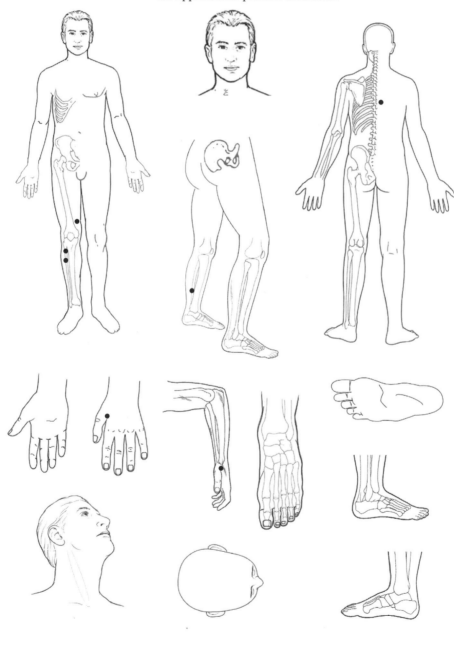

Cramps (Menstrual)

Emergency Nutritional Daily Menu	Maintenance Nutritional Daily Menu
Glyco: 2 tsp Phyto: 1 tsp Pre-Hormone: 6 tabs Essentials: 4 tabs	Glyco: 1 tsp Phyto: 1/2 tsp Pre-Hormone: 4 tabs Essentials: 4 tabs

see appendix for product definitions

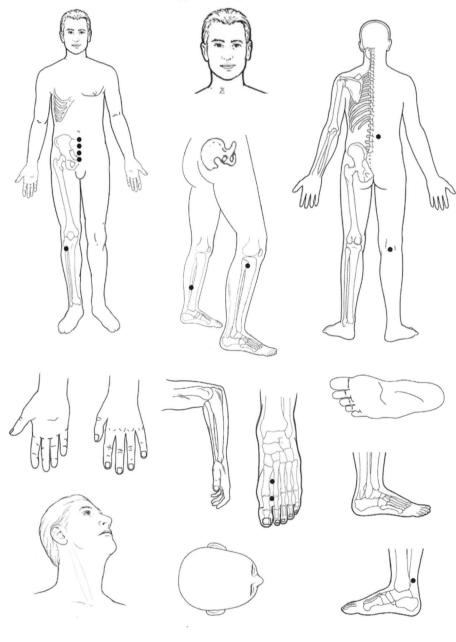

118

Cravings (Sweets/Alcohol)

Emergency Nutritional Daily Menu	Maintenance Nutritional Daily Menu
Glyco: 3 tsp Phyto: 2 tsp Pre-Hormone: 3 tabs Cata-Blend: 4 tabs	Glyco: 1 tsp Phyto: 1 tsp Pre-Hormone: 4 tabs Cata-Blend: 4 tabs

see appendix for product definitions

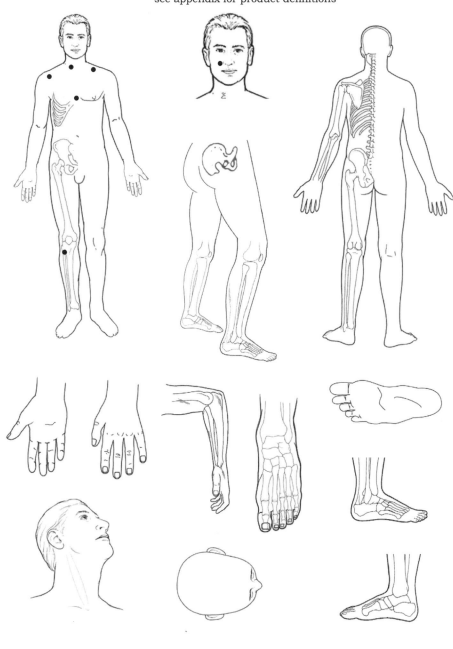

119

Crohn's Disease

Emergency Nutritional Daily Menu	Maintenance Nutritional Daily Menu
Glyco: 6 tsp Phyto: 2 tsp Pre-Hormone: 6 tabs Cata-Blend: 4 tabs	Glyco: 2 tsp Phyto: 1 tsp Pre-Hormone: 4 tabs Cata-Blend: 4 tabs

see appendix for product definitions

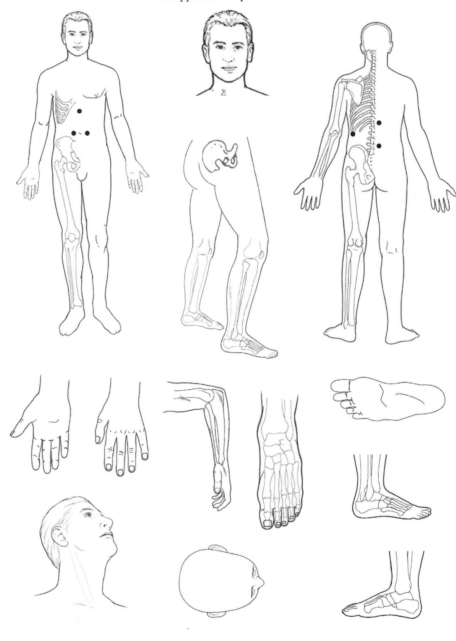

Croup

Emergency Nutritional Daily Menu	Maintenance Nutritional Daily Menu
Glyco: 3 tsp Phyto: 1 tsp Pre-Hormone: 3 tabs Essentials: 4 tabs	Glyco: 1 tsp Phyto: 1/2 tsp Pre-Hormone: 3 tabs Essentials: 4 tabs

see appendix for product definitions

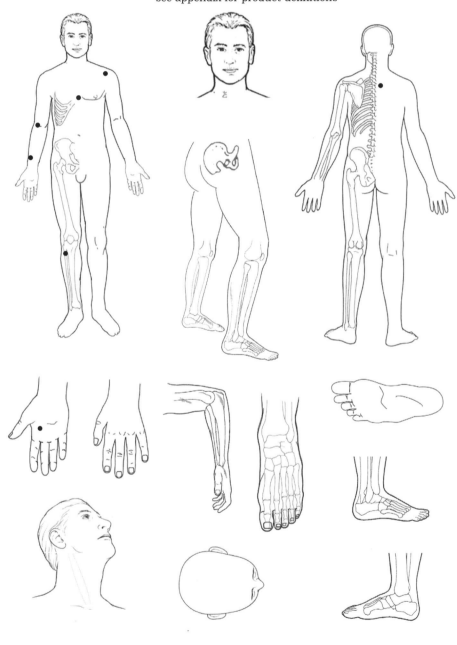

Cushing's Syndrome

Emergency Nutritional Daily Menu	Maintenance Nutritional Daily Menu
Glyco: 3 tsp Phyto: 1 tsp Pre-Hormone: 3 tabs Cata-Blend: 4 tabs	Glyco: 2 tsp Phyto: 1 tsp Pre-Hormone: 3 tabs Cata-Blend: 4 tabs

see appendix for product definitions

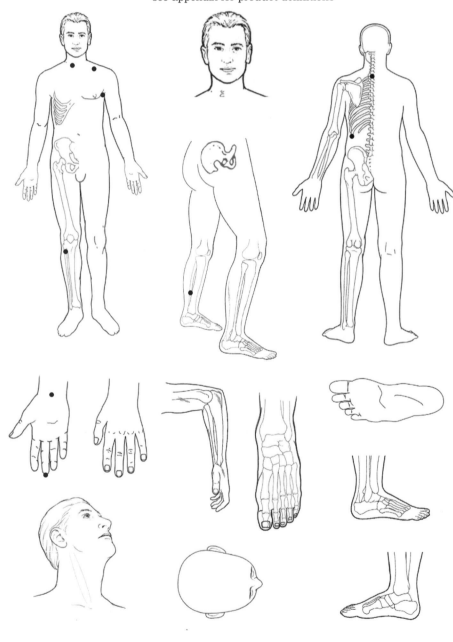

122

CVA / Stroke

Emergency Nutritional Daily Menu	Maintenance Nutritional Daily Menu
Glyco: 6 tsp Phyto: 2 tsp Pre-Hormone: 4 tabs Cata-Blend: 6 tabs	Glyco: 2 tsp Phyto: 1 tsp Pre-Hormone: 3 tabs Cata-Blend: 4 tabs

see appendix for product definitions

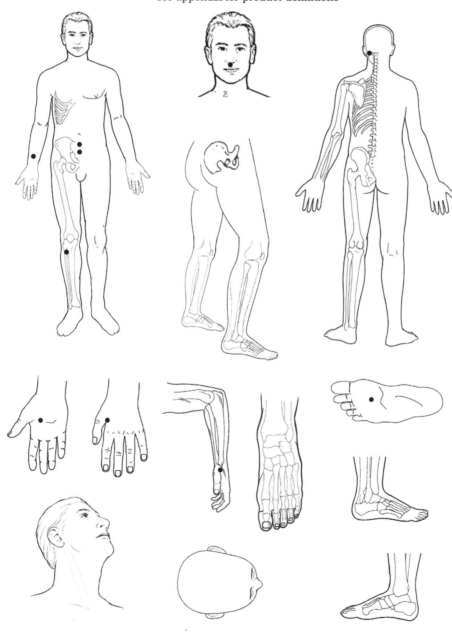

Cystitis (Acute UTI)

Emergency Nutritional Daily Menu	Maintenance Nutritional Daily Menu
Glyco: 3 tsp Phyto: 1 tsp Pre-Hormone: 3 tabs Essentials: 4 tabs	Glyco: NA Phyto: NA Pre-Hormone: 3 tabs Essentials: 4 tabs

see appendix for product definitions

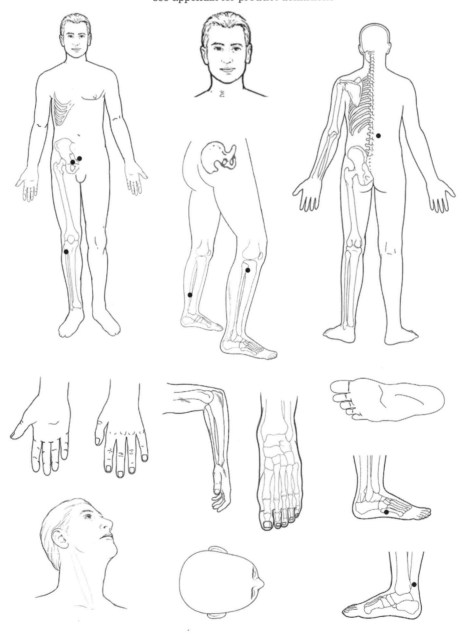

Cystitis (Chronic)

Emergency Nutritional Daily Menu	Maintenance Nutritional Daily Menu
Glyco: 3 tsp Phyto: 1 tsp Pre-Hormone: 3 tabs Essentials: 4 tabs	Glyco: 2 tsp Phyto: 1 tsp Pre-Hormone: 3 tabs Essentials: 4 tabs

see appendix for product definitions

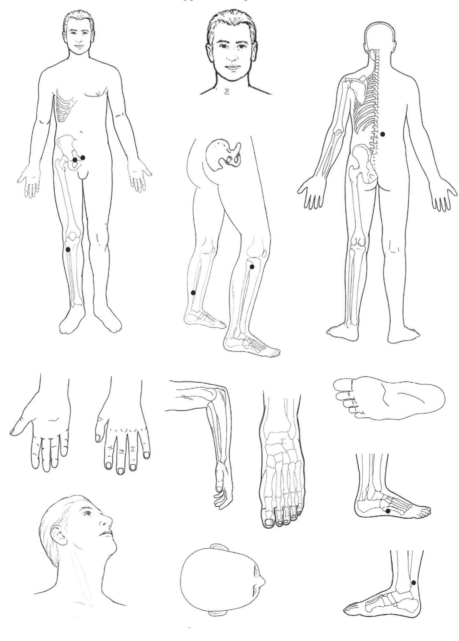

Cysts- Breasts

Emergency Nutritional Daily Menu	Maintenance Nutritional Daily Menu
Glyco: 3 tsp Phyto: 1 tsp Pre-Hormone: 4 tabs Cata-Blend: 4 tabs	Glyco: 2 tsp Phyto: 1 tsp Pre-Hormone: 4 tabs Cata-Blend: 4 tabs

see appendix for product definitions

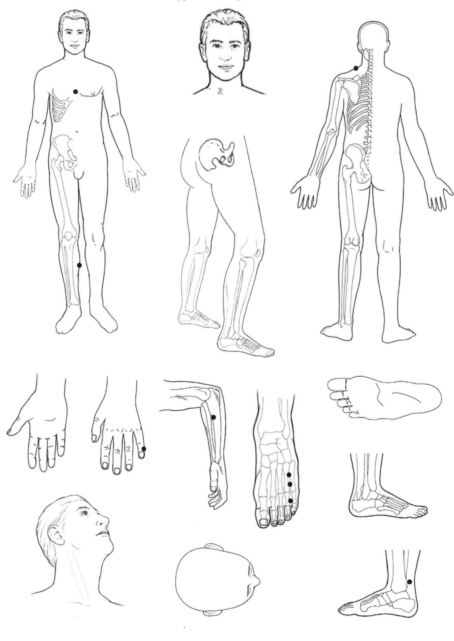

Cytomegalovirus

Emergency Nutritional Daily Menu	Maintenance Nutritional Daily Menu
Glyco: 3 tsp Phyto: 2 tsp Pre-Hormone: 3 tabs Cata-Blend: 6 tabs	Glyco: 2 tsp Phyto: 1 tsp Pre-Hormone: 3 tabs Cata-Blend: 4 tabs

see appendix for product definitions

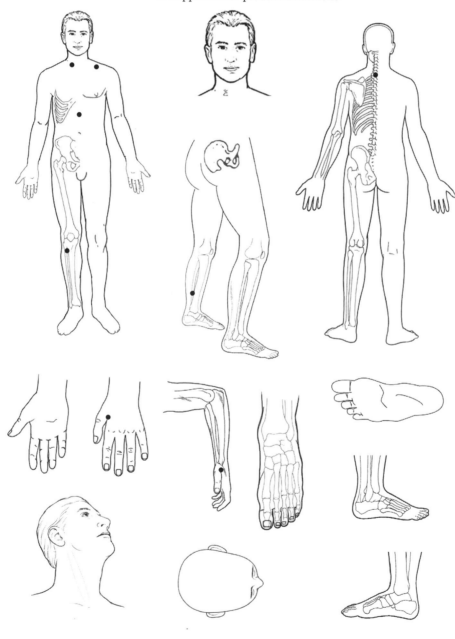

Dandruff

Emergency Nutritional Daily Menu	Maintenance Nutritional Daily Menu
Glyco: 1 tsp Phyto: 1 tsp Pre-Hormone: 3 tabs Essentials: 4 tabs	Glyco: 1/2 tsp Phyto: 1/2 tsp Pre-Hormone: 3 tabs Essentials: 4 tabs

see appendix for product definitions

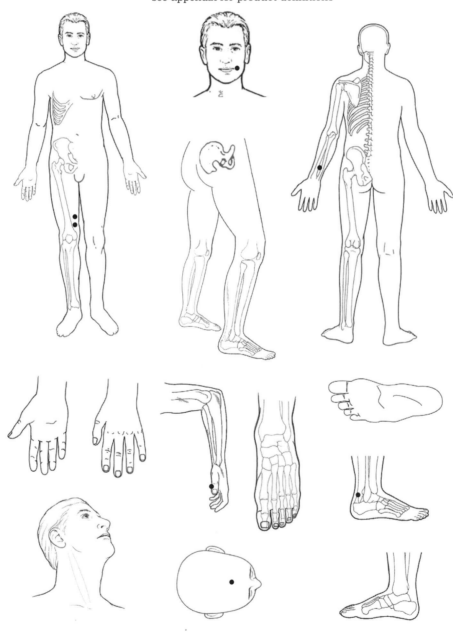

Decubitus Ulcer
(apply soft laser to affect areas)

Emergency Nutritional Daily Menu	Maintenance Nutritional Daily Menu
Glyco: 3 tsp Phyto: 2 tsp Pre-Hormone: 6 tabs Cata-Blend: 6 tabs	Glyco: 1 tsp Phyto: 1 tsp Pre-Hormone: 3 tabs Cata-Blend: 4 tabs

see appendix for product definitions

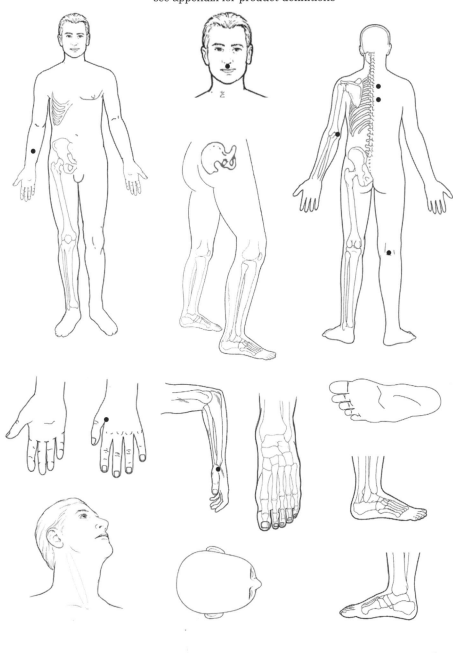

Deep Vein Thrombosis (DVT)

Emergency Nutritional Daily Menu	Maintenance Nutritional Daily Menu
Glyco: 2 tsp Phyto: 1 tsp Pre-Hormone: 3 tabs Essentials: 4 tabs	Glyco: 1 tsp Phyto: 1/2 tsp Pre-Hormone: 3 tabs Essentials: 4 tabs

see appendix for product definitions

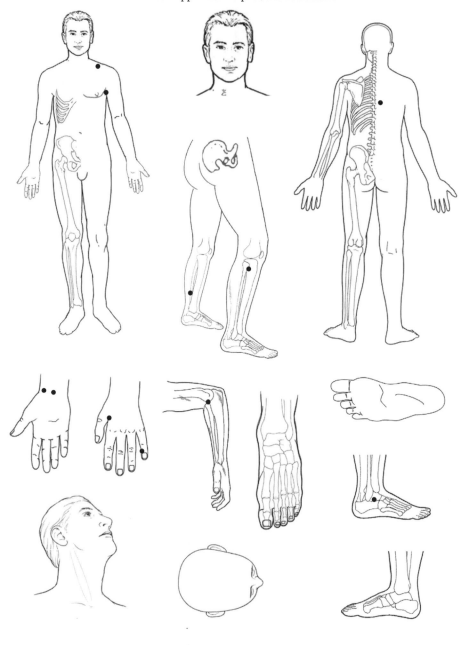

130

Degenerative Disc Disease

Emergency Nutritional Daily Menu	Maintenance Nutritional Daily Menu
Glyco: 3 tsp Phyto: 1 tsp Pre-Hormone: 3 tabs Cata-Blend: 6 tabs	Glyco: 2 tsp Phyto: 1 tsp Pre-Hormone: 3 tabs Cata-Blend: 4 tabs

see appendix for product definitions

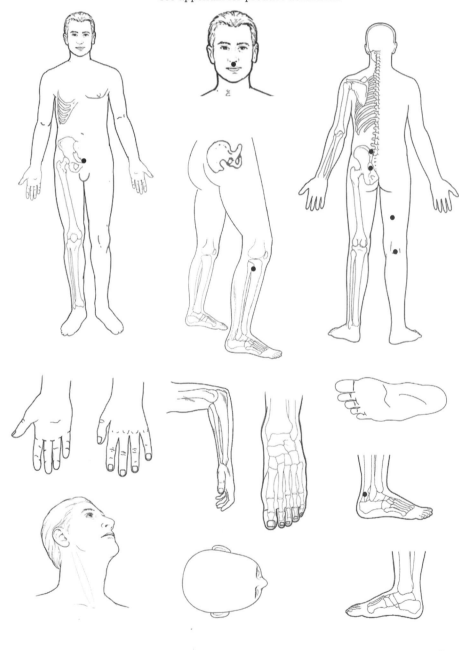

Degenerative Joint Disease (DJD)

Emergency Nutritional Daily Menu	Maintenance Nutritional Daily Menu
Glyco: 4 tsp Phyto: 2 tsp Pre-Hormone: 4 tabs Cata-Blend: 6 tabs	Glyco: 2 tsp Phyto: 1 tsp Pre-Hormone: 3 tabs Cata-Blend: 6 tabs

see appendix for product definitions

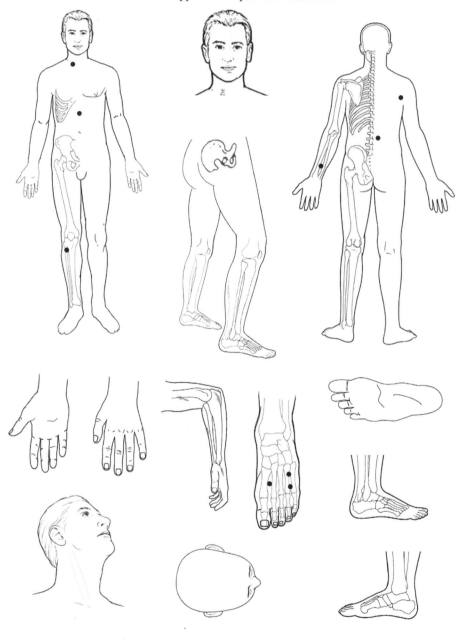

Depression

Emergency Nutritional Daily Menu	Maintenance Nutritional Daily Menu
Glyco: 4 tsp Phyto: 2 tsp Pre-Hormone: 6 tabs Cata-Blend: 4 tabs	Glyco: 2 tsp Phyto: 1 tsp Pre-Hormone: 4 tabs Cata-Blend: 4 tabs

see appendix for product definitions

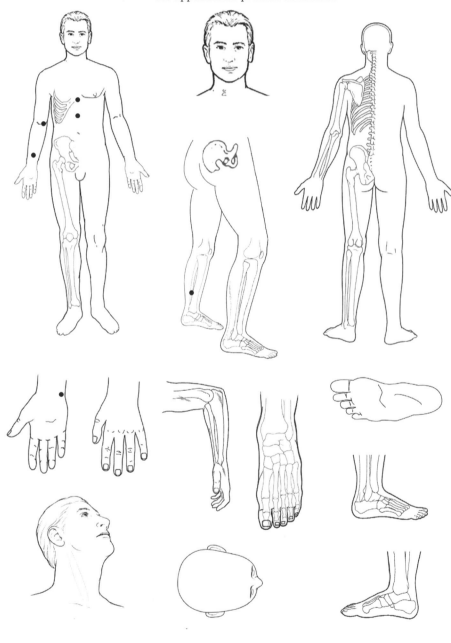

Dermatitis, Atopic Eczema
(apply soft laser to affect areas)

Emergency Nutritional Daily Menu	Maintenance Nutritional Daily Menu
Glyco: 3 tsp Phyto: 2 tsp Pre-Hormone: 3 tabs Essentials: 4 tabs	Glyco: 1 tsp Phyto: 1 tsp Pre-Hormone: 3 tabs Essentials: 4 tabs

see appendix for product definitions

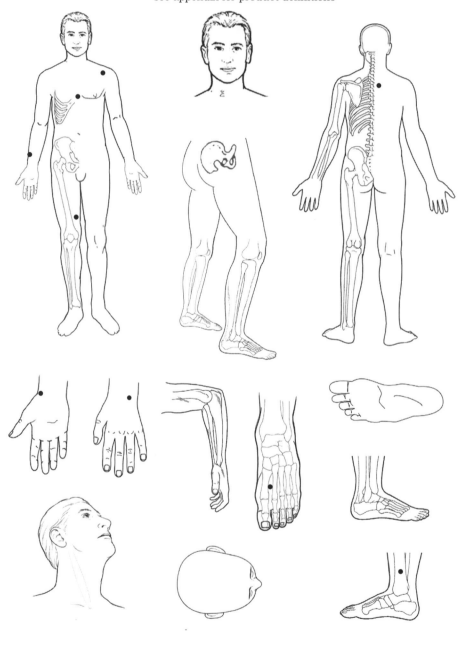

Detoxification (Systemic)

Emergency Nutritional Daily Menu	Maintenance Nutritional Daily Menu
Glyco: 9 tsp Phyto: 2 tsp Pre-Hormone: 4 tabs Cata-Blend: 4 tabs	Glyco: 1/2 tsp Phyto: 1/2 tsp Pre-Hormone: 3 tabs Cata-Blend: 4 tabs

see appendix for product definitions

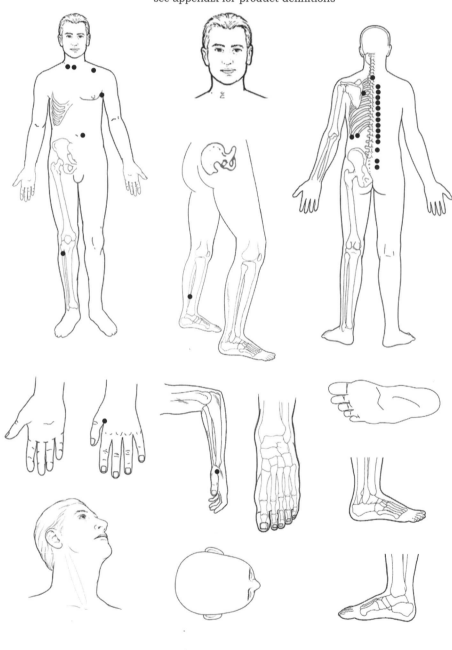

135

Diabetes

Emergency Nutritional Daily Menu	Maintenance Nutritional Daily Menu
Glyco: 3 tsp Phyto: 2 tsp Pre-Hormone: 6 tabs Cata-Blend: 6 tabs	Glyco: 2 tsp Phyto: 2 tsp Pre-Hormone: 6 tabs Cata-Blend: 6 tabs

see appendix for product definitions

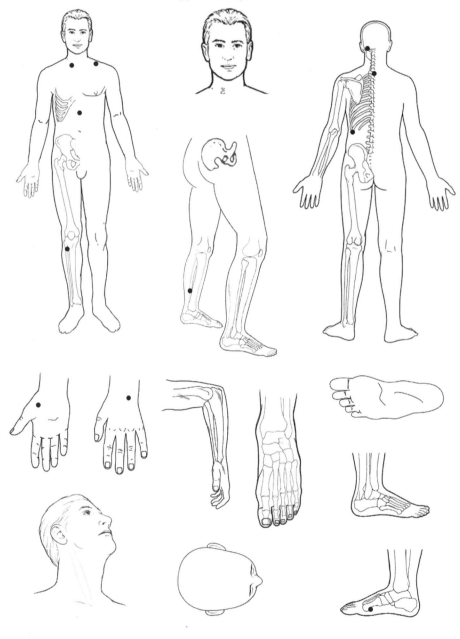

Diabetic Sores
(apply soft laser to affect areas)

Emergency Nutritional Daily Menu	Maintenance Nutritional Daily Menu
Glyco: 3 tsp Phyto: 2 tsp Pre-Hormone: 6 tabs Cata-Blend: 6 tabs	Glyco: 2 tsp Phyto: 1 tsp Pre-Hormone: 3 tabs Cata-Blend: 6 tabs

see appendix for product definitions

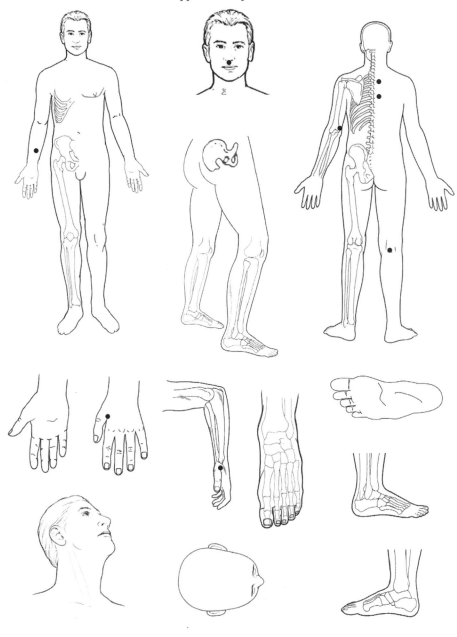

Diarrhea

Emergency Nutritional Daily Menu	Maintenance Nutritional Daily Menu
Glyco: 3 tsp Phyto: 1 tsp Pre-Hormone: 3 tabs Essentials: 4 tabs	Glyco: 1/2 tsp Phyto: 1/2 tsp Pre-Hormone: 3 tabs Essentials: 4 tabs

see appendix for product definitions

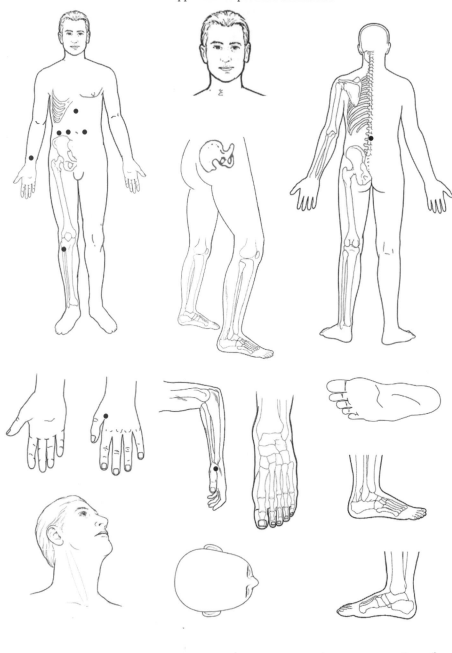

Diverticulitis w/o Hemorrhage

Emergency Nutritional Daily Menu	Maintenance Nutritional Daily Menu
Glyco: 3 tsp Phyto: 2 tsp Pre-Hormone: 3 tabs Cata-Blend: 4 tabs	Glyco: 1 tsp Phyto: 1 tsp Pre-Hormone: 3 tabs Cata-Blend: 4 tabs

see appendix for product definitions

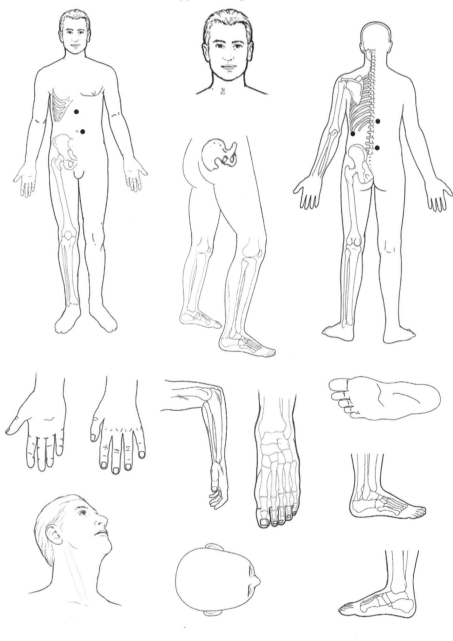

139

Dizziness (Vertigo)

Emergency Nutritional Daily Menu	Maintenance Nutritional Daily Menu
Glyco: 3 tsp Phyto: 1 tsp Pre-Hormone: 3 tabs Cata-Blend: 4 tabs	Glyco: 1/2 tsp Phyto: 1/2 tsp Pre-Hormone: 3 tabs Cata-Blend: 4 tabs

see appendix for product definitions

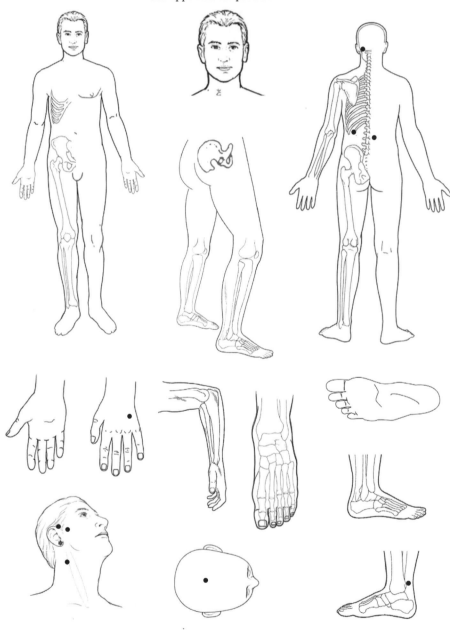

140

DJD (Degenerative Joint Disease)

Emergency Nutritional Daily Menu	Maintenance Nutritional Daily Menu
Glyco: 3 tsp Phyto: 1 tsp Pre-Hormone: 4 tabs Cata-Blend: 6 tabs	Glyco: 2 tsp Phyto: 1 tsp Pre-Hormone: 4 tabs Cata-Blend: 4 tabs

see appendix for product definitions

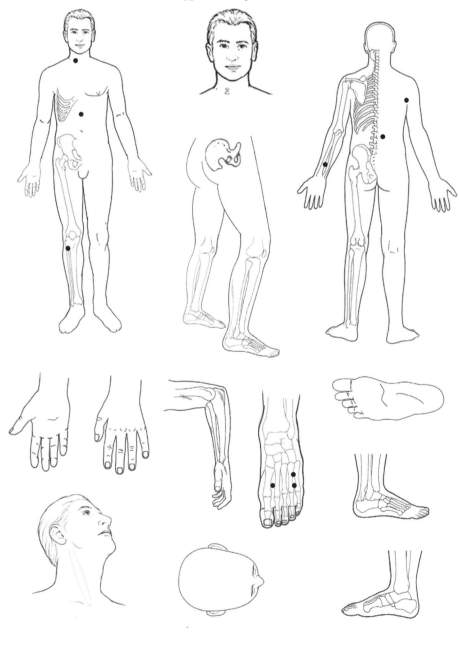

141

Drug Addiction

Emergency Nutritional Daily Menu	Maintenance Nutritional Daily Menu
Glyco: 4 tsp Phyto: 1 tsp Pre-Hormone: 6 tabs Cata-Blend: 6 tabs	Glyco: 2 tsp Phyto: 1 tsp Pre-Hormone: 4 tabs Cata-Blend: 4 tabs

see appendix for product definitions

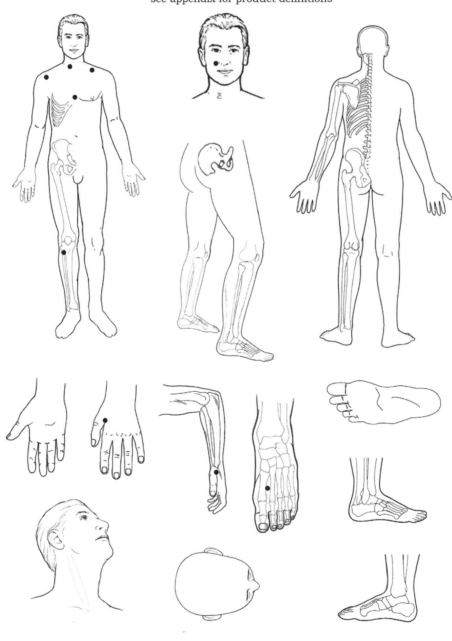

Duodenal Ulcer

Emergency Nutritional Daily Menu	Maintenance Nutritional Daily Menu
Glyco: 3 tsp Phyto: 1 tsp Pre-Hormone: 3 tabs Cata-Blend: 4 tabs	Glyco: 1 tsp Phyto: 1 tsp Pre-Hormone: 3 tabs Cata-Blend: 4 tabs

see appendix for product definitions

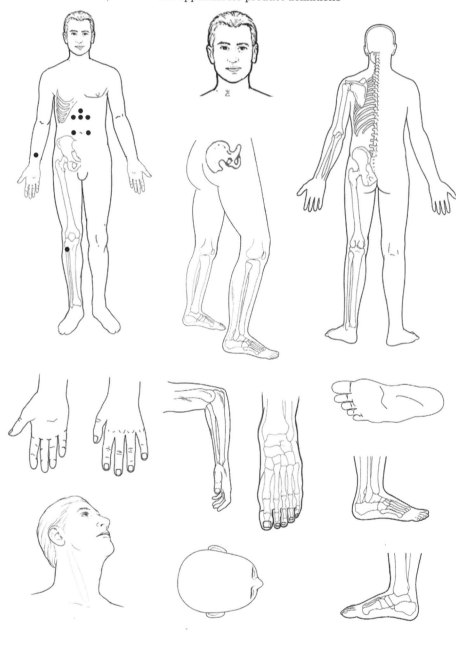

DVT (Deep Vein Thrombosis)

Emergency Nutritional Daily Menu	Maintenance Nutritional Daily Menu
Glyco: 2 tsp Phyto: 1 tsp Pre-Hormone: 3 tabs Essentials: 4 tabs	Glyco: 1 tsp Phyto: 1/2 tsp Pre-Hormone: 3 tabs Essentials: 4 tabs

see appendix for product definitions

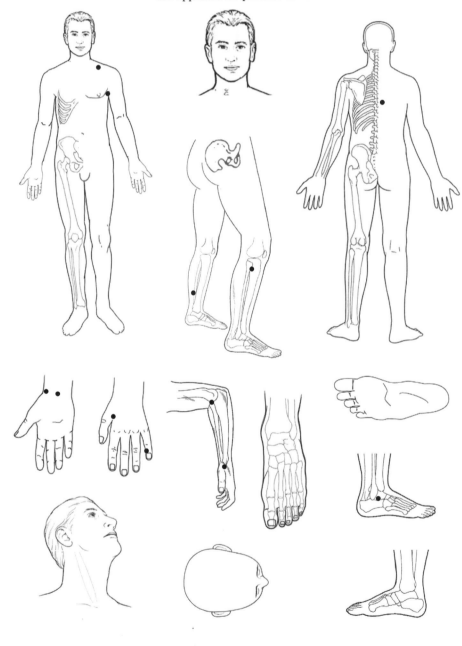

Dyslexia

Emergency Nutritional Daily Menu	Maintenance Nutritional Daily Menu
Glyco: 6 tsp Phyto: 2 tsp Pre-Hormone: 6 tabs Cata-Blend: 6 tabs	Glyco: 2 tsp Phyto: 1 tsp Pre-Hormone: 3 tabs Cata-Blend: 4 tabs

see appendix for product definitions

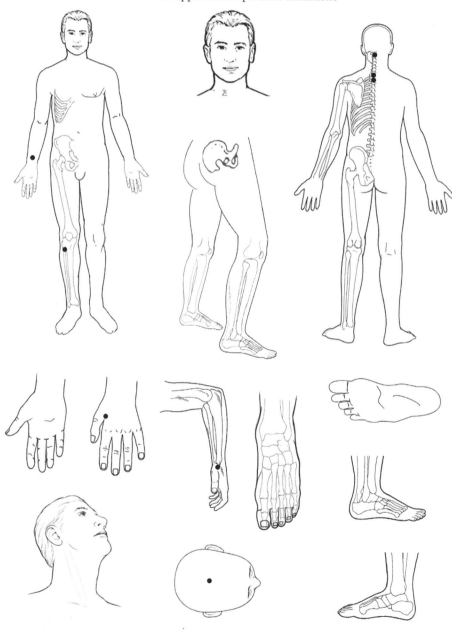

Dyspepsia

Emergency Nutritional Daily Menu	Maintenance Nutritional Daily Menu
Glyco: 3 tsp Phyto: 1 tsp Pre-Hormone: 4 tabs Essentials: 6 tabs	Glyco: 1 tsp Phyto: 1/2 tsp Pre-Hormone: 3 tabs Essentials: 4 tabs

see appendix for product definitions

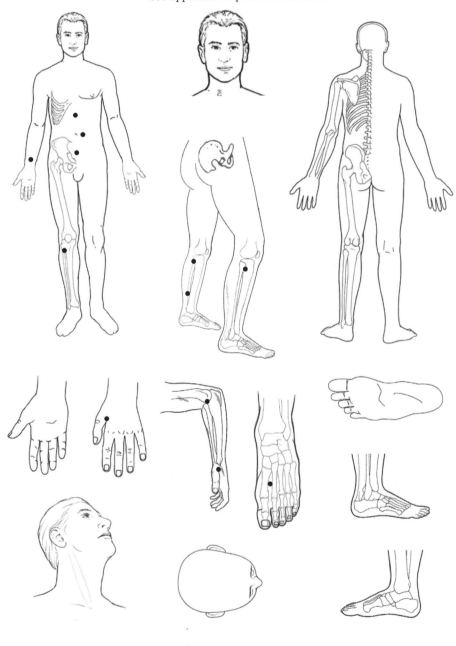

146

Dyspnea

Emergency Nutritional Daily Menu	Maintenance Nutritional Daily Menu
Glyco: 3 tsp Phyto: 1 tsp Pre-Hormone: 3 tabs Essentials: 4 tabs	Glyco: 1 tsp Phyto: 1/2 tsp Pre-Hormone: 3 tabs Essentials: 4 tabs

see appendix for product definitions

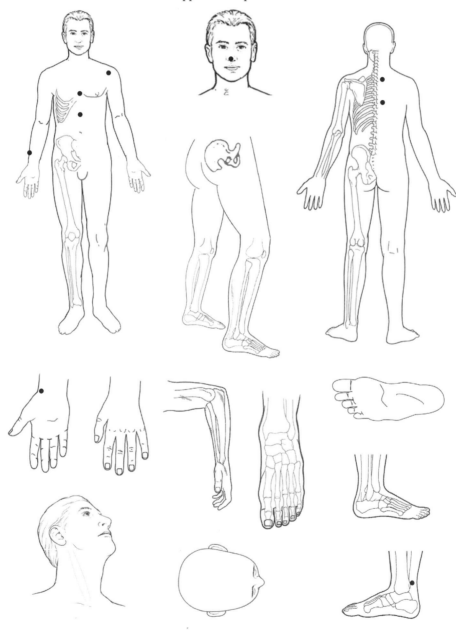

Dysuria

Emergency Nutritional Daily Menu	Maintenance Nutritional Daily Menu
Glyco: 3 tsp Phyto: 1 tsp Pre-Hormone: 3 tabs Essentials: 4 tabs	Glyco: 1 tsp Phyto: 1/2 tsp Pre-Hormone: 3 tabs Essentials: 4 tabs

see appendix for product definitions

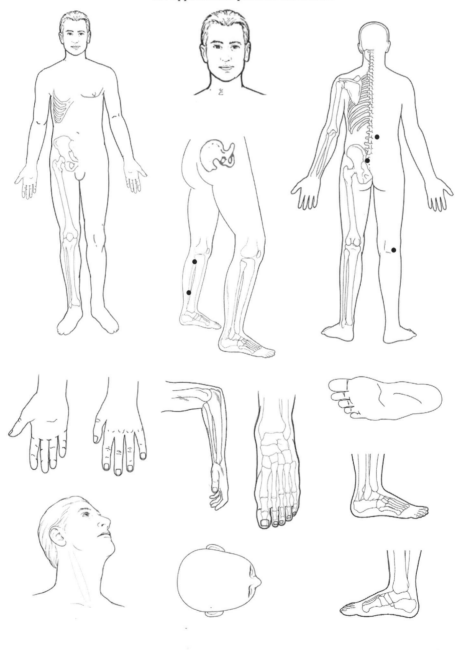

Earache

Emergency Nutritional Daily Menu	Maintenance Nutritional Daily Menu
Glyco: 3 tsp Phyto: 1 tsp Pre-Hormone: 3 tabs Essentials: 4 tabs	Glyco: 1/2 tsp Phyto: 1/2 tsp Pre-Hormone: 3 tabs Essentials: 4 tabs

see appendix for product definitions

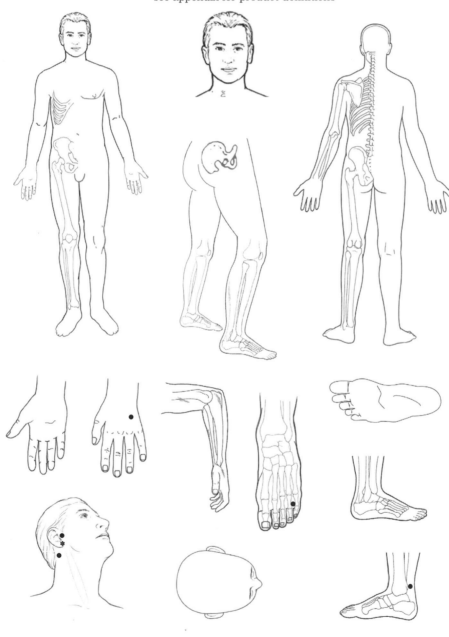

Elevated Blood Pressure w/o Hypertension

Emergency Nutritional Daily Menu	Maintenance Nutritional Daily Menu
Glyco: 3 tsp Phyto: 2 tsp Pre-Hormone: 6 tabs Cata-Blend: 4 tabs	Glyco: 1 tsp Phyto: 1 tsp Pre-Hormone: 4 tabs Cata-Blend: 4 tabs

see appendix for product definitions

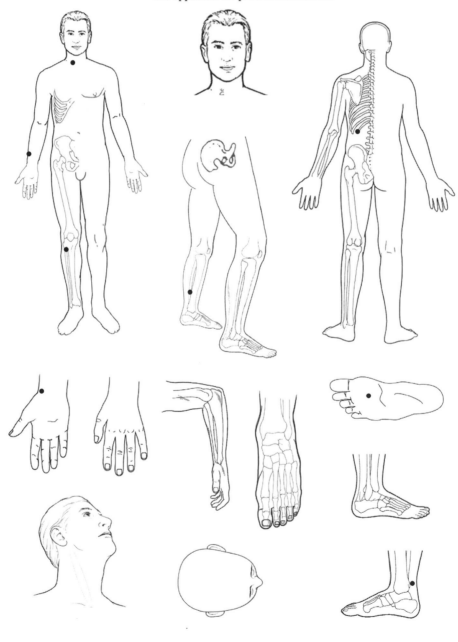

150

Emphysema

Emergency Nutritional Daily Menu	Maintenance Nutritional Daily Menu
Glyco: 3 tsp Phyto: 2 tsp Pre-Hormone: 3 tabs Cata-Blend: 4 tabs	Glyco: 2 tsp Phyto: 1 tsp Pre-Hormone: 3 tabs Cata-Blend: 4 tabs

see appendix for product definitions

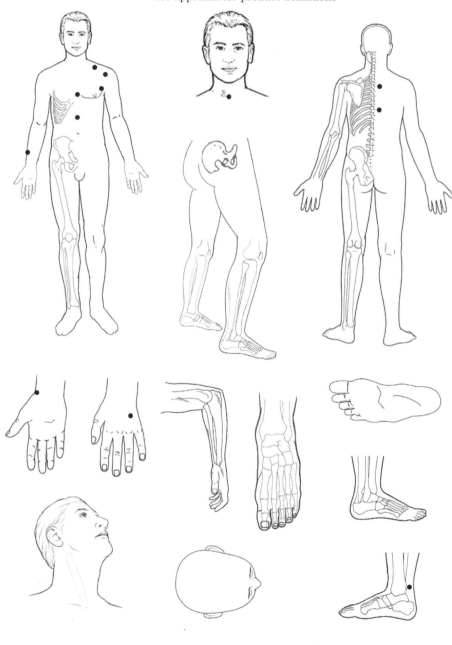

Endocarditis (Acute/Subacute Bacterial)

Emergency Nutritional Daily Menu	Maintenance Nutritional Daily Menu
Glyco: 6 tsp Phyto: 2 tsp Pre-Hormone: 3 tabs Cata-Blend: 6 tabs	Glyco: 2 tsp Phyto: 1 tsp Pre-Hormone: 3 tabs Cata-Blend: 4 tabs

see appendix for product definitions

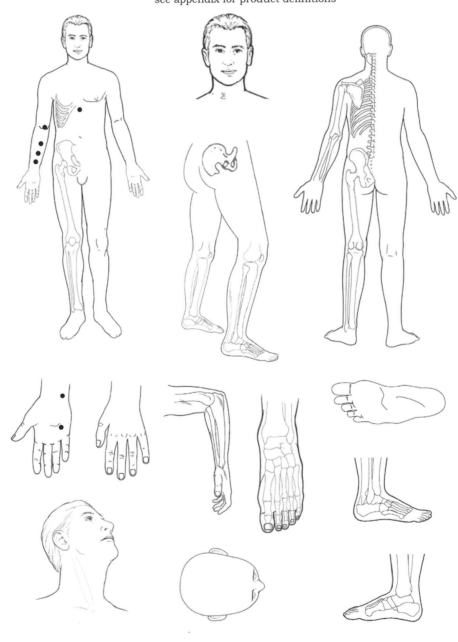

Endocervicitis

Emergency Nutritional Daily Menu	Maintenance Nutritional Daily Menu
Glyco: 3 tsp Phyto: 1 tsp Pre-Hormone: 3 tabs Cata-Blend: 4 tabs	Glyco: 1 tsp Phyto: 1 tsp Pre-Hormone: 3 tabs Cata-Blend: 4 tabs

see appendix for product definitions

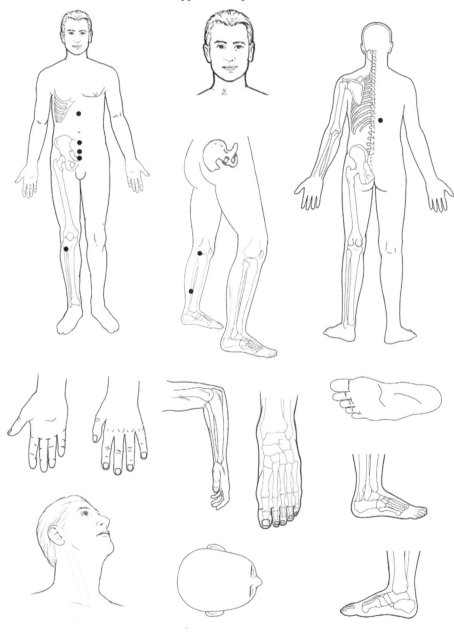

Endometriosis

Emergency Nutritional Daily Menu	Maintenance Nutritional Daily Menu
Glyco: 3 tsp Phyto: 1 tsp Pre-Hormone: 3 tabs Cata-Blend: 4 tabs	Glyco: 2 tsp Phyto: 1 tsp Pre-Hormone: 3 tabs Cata-Blend: 4 tabs

see appendix for product definitions

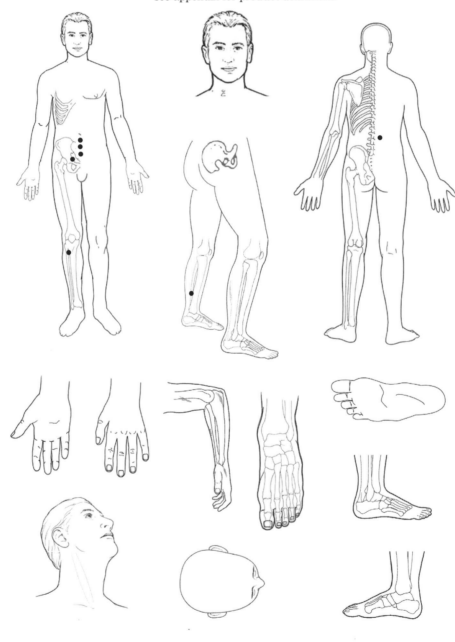

154

Enteritis (Bacterial)

Emergency Nutritional Daily Menu	Maintenance Nutritional Daily Menu
Glyco: 3 tsp Phyto: 1 tsp Pre-Hormone: 3 tabs Cata-Blend: 4 tabs	Glyco: 1/2 tsp Phyto: 1/2 tsp Pre-Hormone: 3 tabs Cata-Blend: 4 tabs

see appendix for product definitions

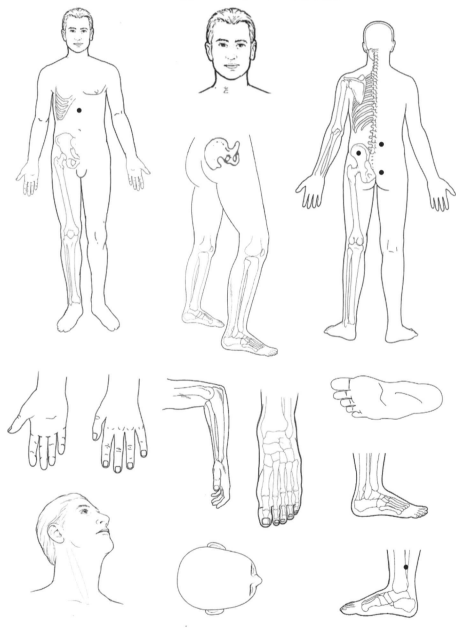

Enterocolitis, Ulcerative, Chronic

Emergency Nutritional Daily Menu	Maintenance Nutritional Daily Menu
Glyco: 9 tsp Phyto: 2 tsp Pre-Hormone: 3 tabs Cata-Blend: 4 tabs	Glyco: 2 tsp Phyto: 1 tsp Pre-Hormone: 3 tabs Cata-Blend: 4 tabs

see appendix for product definitions

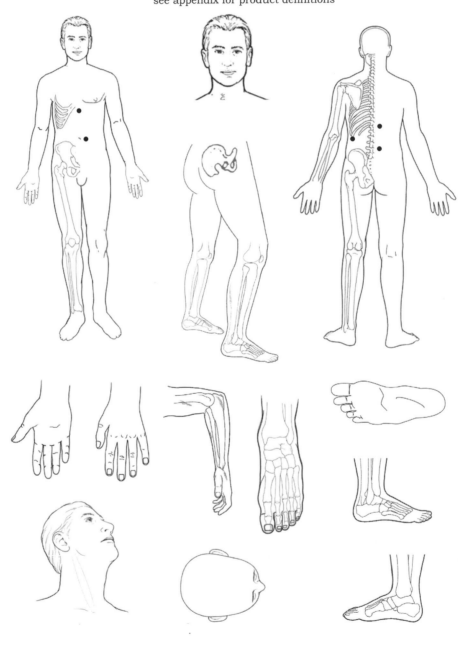

Epstein-Barr Virus

Emergency Nutritional Daily Menu	Maintenance Nutritional Daily Menu
Glyco: 6 tsp Phyto: 2 tsp Pre-Hormone: 3 tabs Cata-Blend: 6 tabs	Glyco: 2 tsp Phyto: 1 tsp Pre-Hormone: 3 tabs Cata-Blend: 4 tabs

see appendix for product definitions

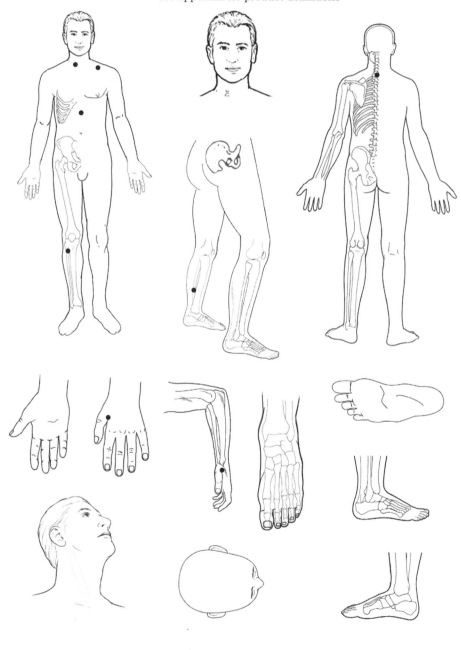

157

Esophageal Spasm

Emergency Nutritional Daily Menu	Maintenance Nutritional Daily Menu
Glyco: 3 tsp Phyto: 1 tsp Pre-Hormone: 3 tabs Essentials: 4 tabs	Glyco: 1 tsp Phyto: 1 tsp Pre-Hormone: 3 tabs Essentials: 4 tabs

see appendix for product definitions

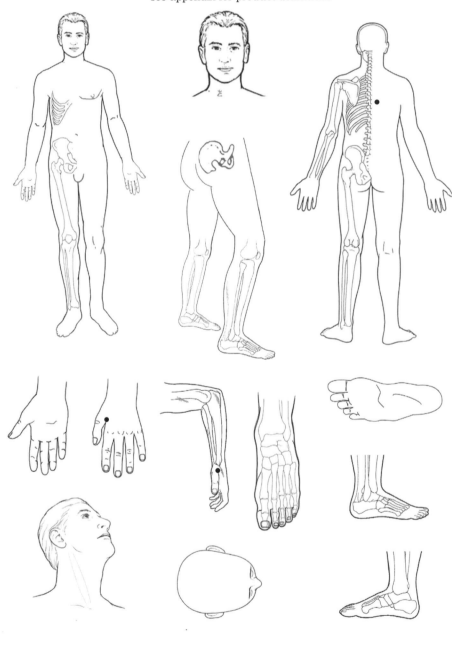

Esophagitis

Emergency Nutritional Daily Menu	Maintenance Nutritional Daily Menu
Glyco: 3 tsp Phyto: 1 tsp Pre-Hormone: 3 tabs Cata-Blend: 4 tabs	Glyco: 1 tsp Phyto: 1/2 tsp Pre-Hormone: 3 tabs Cata-Blend: 4 tabs

see appendix for product definitions

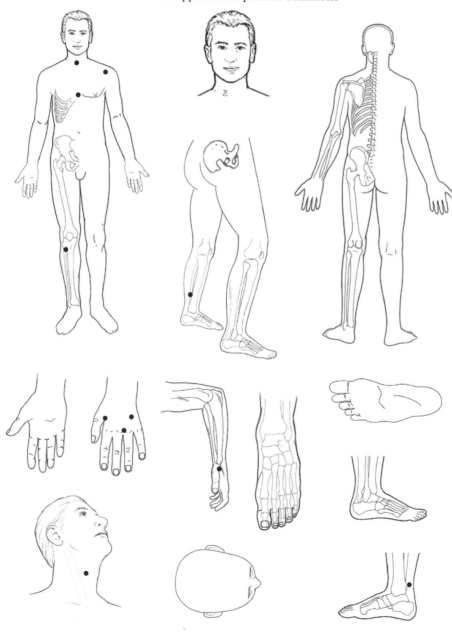

Eustachian Tube Infection

Emergency Nutritional Daily Menu	Maintenance Nutritional Daily Menu
Glyco: 1 tsp Phyto: 1 tsp Pre-Hormone: 3 tabs Essentials: 4 tabs	Glyco: 1/2 tsp Phyto: 1/2 tsp Pre-Hormone: 3 tabs Essentials: 4 tabs

see appendix for product definitions

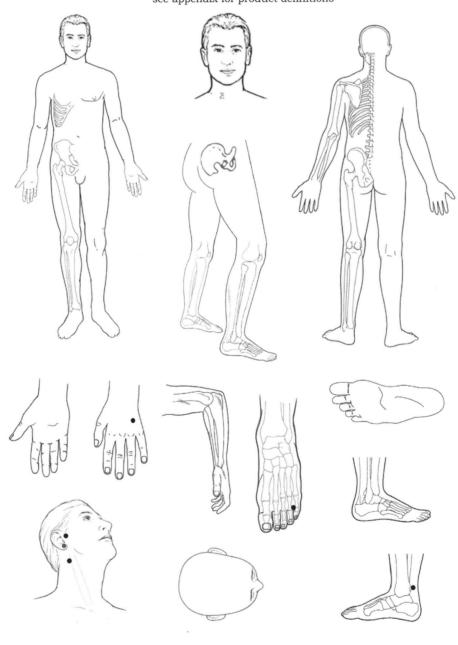

Excessive Sweating (Hyperhidrosis)

Emergency Nutritional Daily Menu	Maintenance Nutritional Daily Menu
Glyco: 3 tsp Phyto: 1 tsp Pre-Hormone: 4 tabs Essentials: 4 tabs	Glyco: 1 tsp Phyto: 1/2 tsp Pre-Hormone: 3 tabs Essentials: 4 tabs

see appendix for product definitions

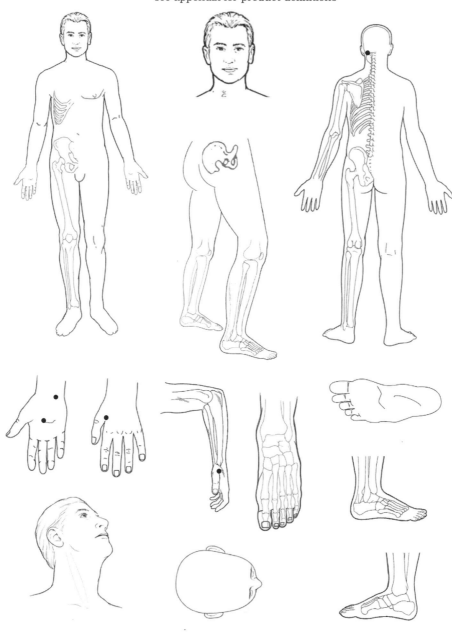

Exercise Intolerance

Emergency Nutritional Daily Menu	Maintenance Nutritional Daily Menu
Glyco: 3 tsp Phyto: 1 tsp Pre-Hormone: 4 tabs Cata-Blend: 4 tabs	Glyco: 1 tsp Phyto: 1/2 tsp Pre-Hormone: 4 tabs Cata-Blend: 4 tabs

see appendix for product definitions

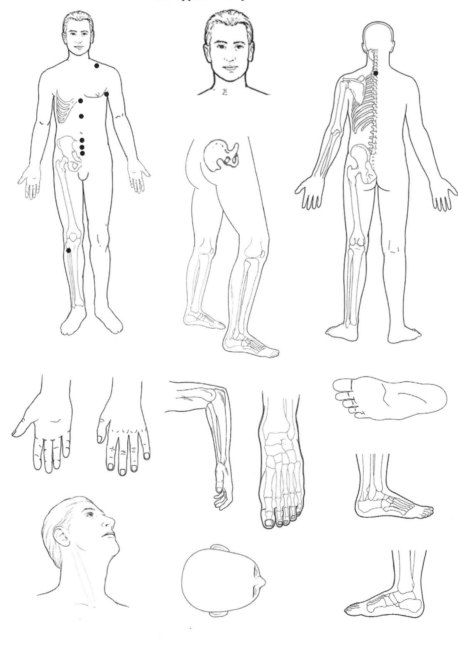

Eyes (Swollen)

Emergency Nutritional Daily Menu	Maintenance Nutritional Daily Menu
Glyco: 3 tsp Phyto: 1 tsp Pre-Hormone: 3 tabs Essentials: 4 tabs	Glyco: 1/2 tsp Phyto: 1/2 tsp Pre-Hormone: 3 tabs Essentials: 4 tabs

see appendix for product definitions

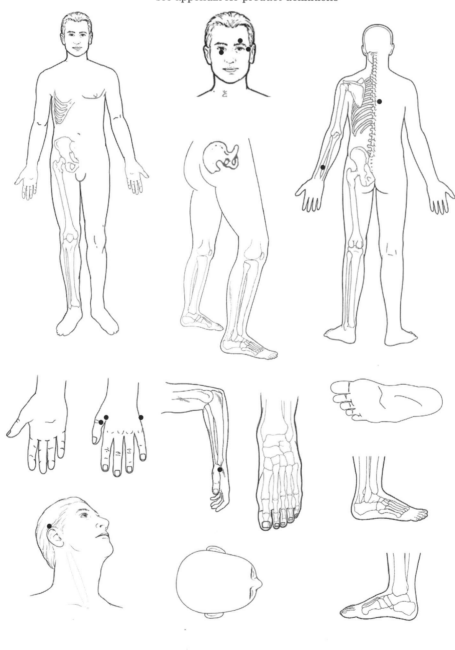

163

Failure to Thrive

Emergency Nutritional Daily Menu	Maintenance Nutritional Daily Menu
Glyco: 6 tsp Phyto: 1 tsp Pre-Hormone: 3 tabs Cata-Blend: 4 tabs	Glyco: 2 tsp Phyto: 1 tsp Pre-Hormone: 3 tabs Cata-Blend: 4 tabs

see appendix for product definitions

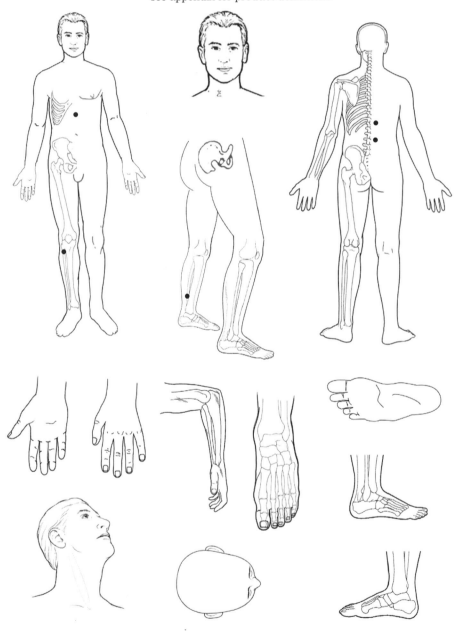

Family History of Breast Cancer

Emergency Nutritional Daily Menu	Maintenance Nutritional Daily Menu
Glyco: 2 tsp Phyto: 1 tsp Pre-Hormone: 3 tabs Cata-Blend: 4 tabs	Glyco: 1 tsp Phyto: 1 tsp Pre-Hormone: 3 tabs Cata-Blend: 4 tabs

see appendix for product definitions

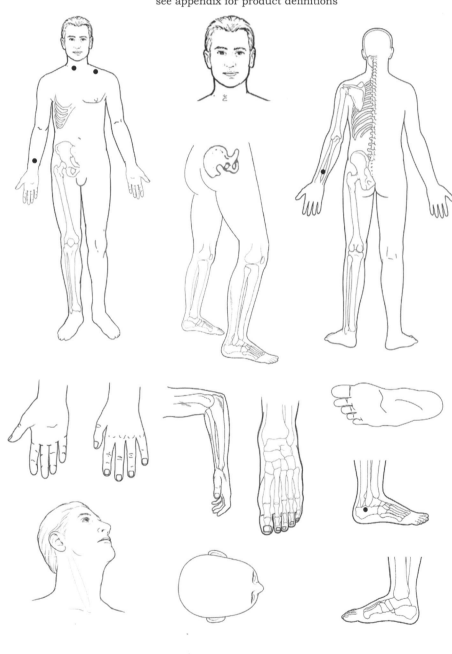

Family History of Coronary Disease

Emergency Nutritional Daily Menu	Maintenance Nutritional Daily Menu
Glyco: 2 tsp Phyto: 1 tsp Pre-Hormone: 3 tabs Cata-Blend: 4 tabs	Glyco: 1 tsp Phyto: 1 tsp Pre-Hormone: 3 tabs Cata-Blend: 4 tabs

see appendix for product definitions

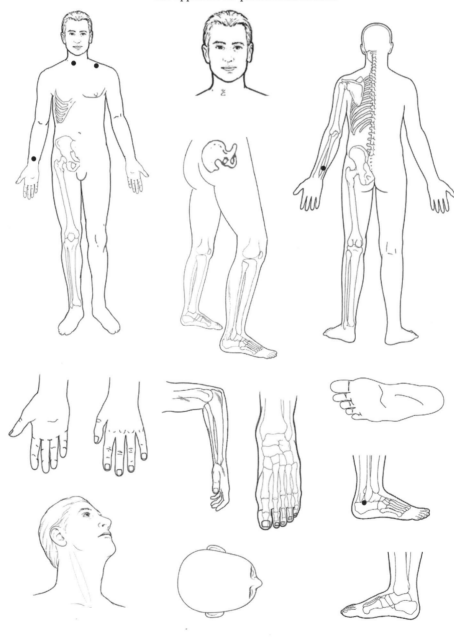

Family History of Diabetes

Emergency Nutritional Daily Menu	Maintenance Nutritional Daily Menu
Glyco: 3 tsp Phyto: 2 tsp Pre-Hormone: 3 tabs Cata-Blend: 4 tabs	Glyco: 1 tsp Phyto: 1 tsp Pre-Hormone: 3 tabs Cata-Blend: 4 tabs

see appendix for product definitions

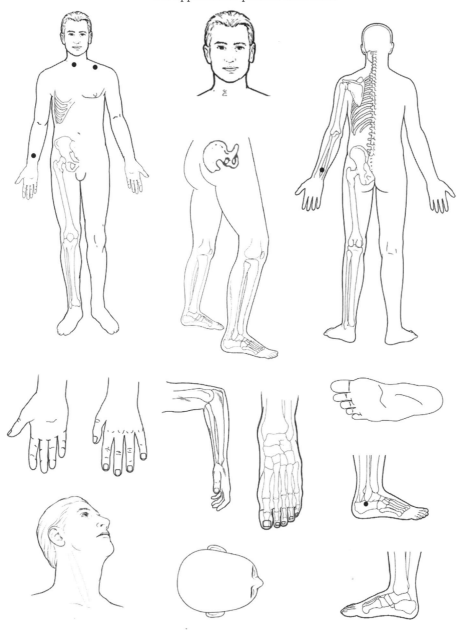

167

Family History of Gastrointestinal Malignancy

Emergency Nutritional Daily Menu	Maintenance Nutritional Daily Menu
Glyco: 3 tsp Phyto: 1 tsp Pre-Hormone: 3 tabs Cata-Blend: 4 tabs	Glyco: 1 tsp Phyto: 1 tsp Pre-Hormone: 3 tabs Cata-Blend: 4 tabs

see appendix for product definitions

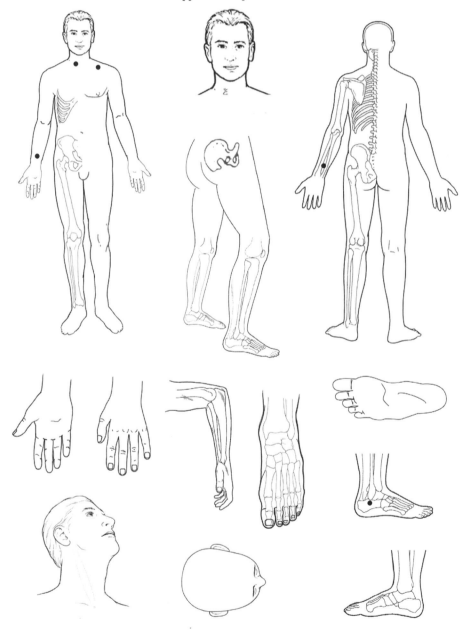

168

Fasciitis

Emergency Nutritional Daily Menu	Maintenance Nutritional Daily Menu
Glyco: 9 tsp Phyto: 1 tsp Pre-Hormone: 6 tabs Cata-Blend: 6 tabs	Glyco: 2 tsp Phyto: 1 tsp Pre-Hormone: 4 tabs Cata-Blend: 4 tabs

see appendix for product definitions

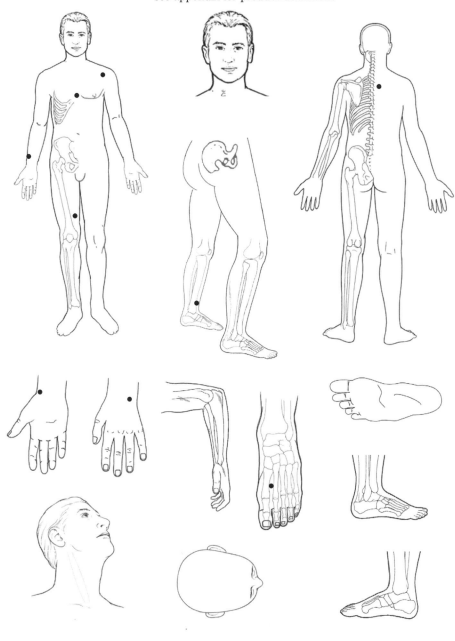

Fatigue/Malaise

Emergency Nutritional Daily Menu	Maintenance Nutritional Daily Menu
Glyco: 6 tsp Phyto: 1 tsp Pre-Hormone: 6 tabs Cata-Blend: 6 tabs	Glyco: 2 tsp Phyto: 1 tsp Pre-Hormone: 4 tabs Cata-Blend: 4 tabs

see appendix for product definitions

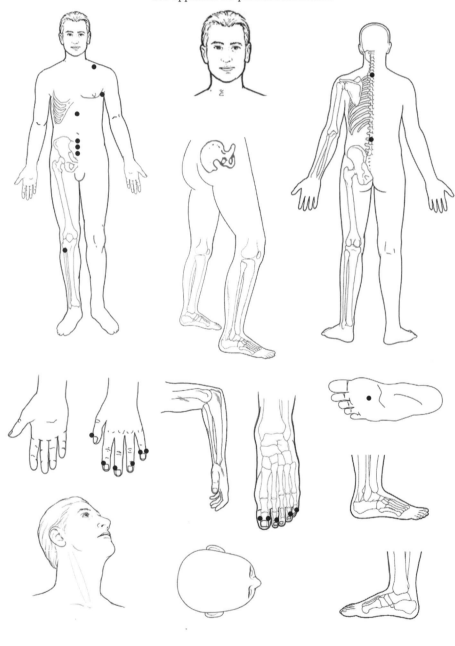

Fever

Emergency Nutritional Daily Menu	Maintenance Nutritional Daily Menu
Glyco: 3 tsp Phyto: 1 tsp Pre-Hormone: 3 tabs Essentials: 4 tabs	Glyco: 1/2 tsp Phyto: 1/2 tsp Pre-Hormone: 3 tabs Essentials: 4 tabs

see appendix for product definitions

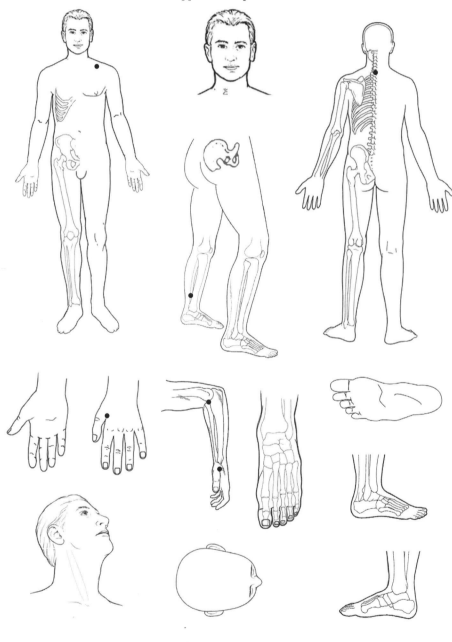

Fibrocystic Breast Disease

Emergency Nutritional Daily Menu	Maintenance Nutritional Daily Menu
Glyco: 3 tsp Phyto: 1 tsp Pre-Hormone: 6 tabs Cata-Blend: 4 tabs	Glyco: 2 tsp Phyto: 1 tsp Pre-Hormone: 4 tabs Cata-Blend: 4 tabs

see appendix for product definitions

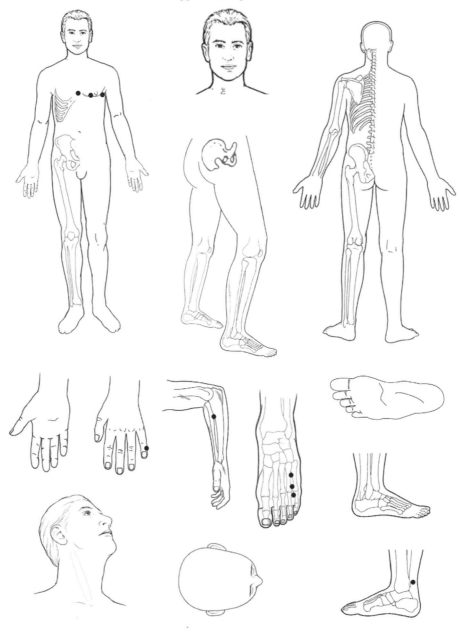

Fibroids (Uterine)

Emergency Nutritional Daily Menu	Maintenance Nutritional Daily Menu
Glyco: 3 tsp Phyto: 1 tsp Pre-Hormone: 6 tabs Cata-Blend: 4 tabs	Glyco: 1 tsp Phyto: 1 tsp Pre-Hormone: 4 tabs Cata-Blend: 4 tabs

see appendix for product definitions

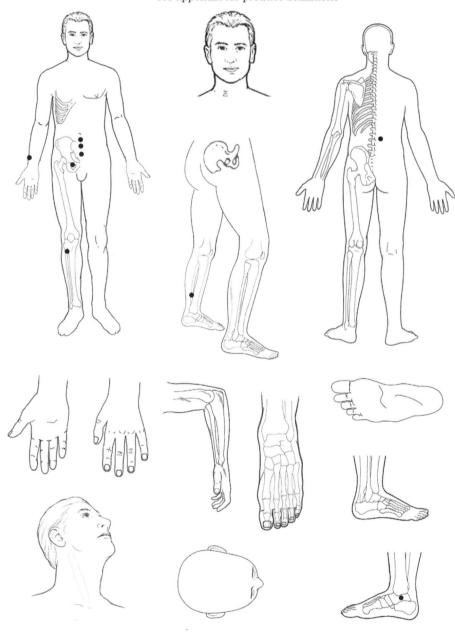

Fibromyalgia

Emergency Nutritional Daily Menu	Maintenance Nutritional Daily Menu
Glyco: 6 tsp Phyto: 2 tsp Pre-Hormone: 6 tabs Cata-Blend: 6 tabs	Glyco: 2 tsp Phyto: 1 tsp Pre-Hormone: 4 tabs Cata-Blend: 4 tabs

see appendix for product definitions

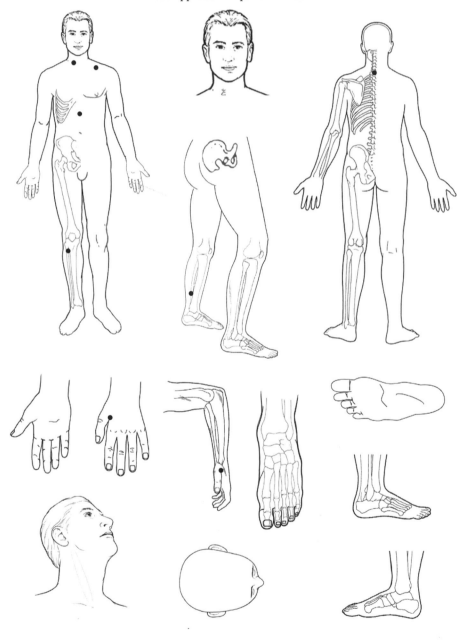

Fibrositis

Emergency Nutritional Daily Menu	Maintenance Nutritional Daily Menu
Glyco: 6 tsp Phyto: 2 tsp Pre-Hormone: 6 tabs Cata-Blend: 6 tabs	Glyco: 2 tsp Phyto: 1 tsp Pre-Hormone: 4 tabs Cata-Blend: 4 tabs

see appendix for product definitions

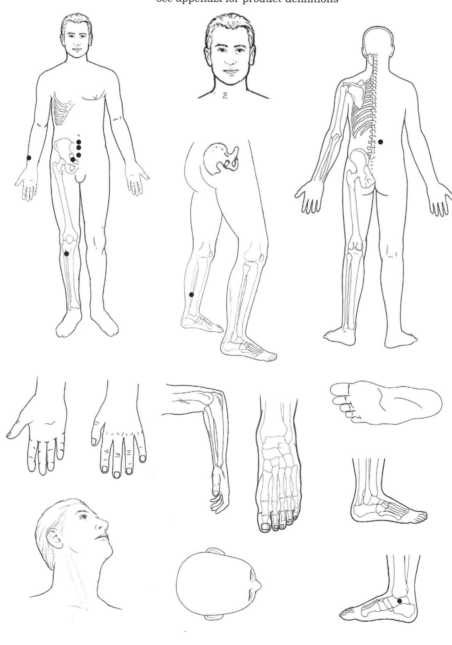

Flatulence

Emergency Nutritional Daily Menu	Maintenance Nutritional Daily Menu
Glyco: 3 tsp Phyto: 1 tsp Pre-Hormone: 3 tabs Essentials: 4 tabs	Glyco: 1 tsp Phyto: 1/2 tsp Pre-Hormone: 3 tabs Essentials: 4 tabs

see appendix for product definitions

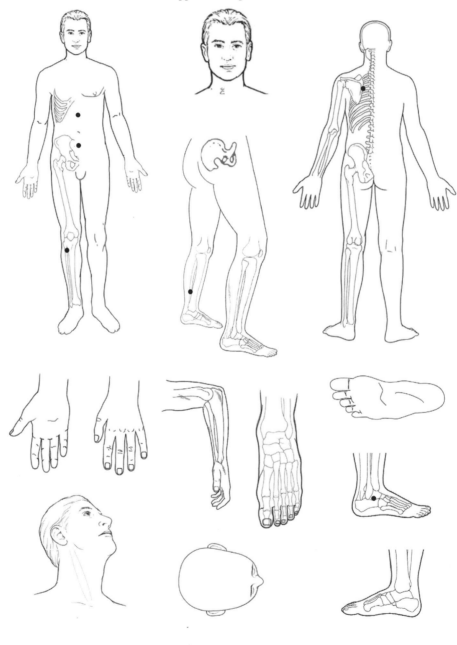

Flora- Restoration Post Antibiotic Therapy

Emergency Nutritional Daily Menu	Maintenance Nutritional Daily Menu
Glyco: 6 tsp Phyto: 2 tsp Pre-Hormone: 3 tabs Essentials: 4 tabs	Glyco: 1/2 tsp Phyto: 1/2 tsp Pre-Hormone: 3 tabs Essentials: 4 tabs

see appendix for product definitions

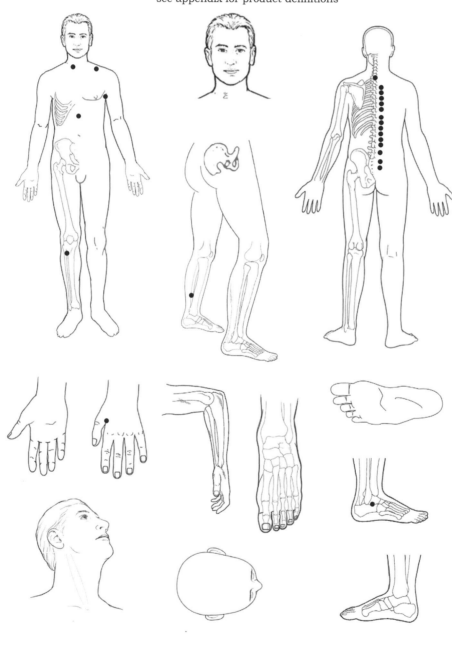

Flu Shot Vaccine

Emergency Nutritional Daily Menu	Maintenance Nutritional Daily Menu
Glyco: 3 tsp Phyto: 1 tsp Pre-Hormone: 3 tabs Essentials: 4 tabs	Glyco: 1/2 tsp Phyto: 1/2 tsp Pre-Hormone: 3 tabs Essentials: 4 tabs

see appendix for product definitions

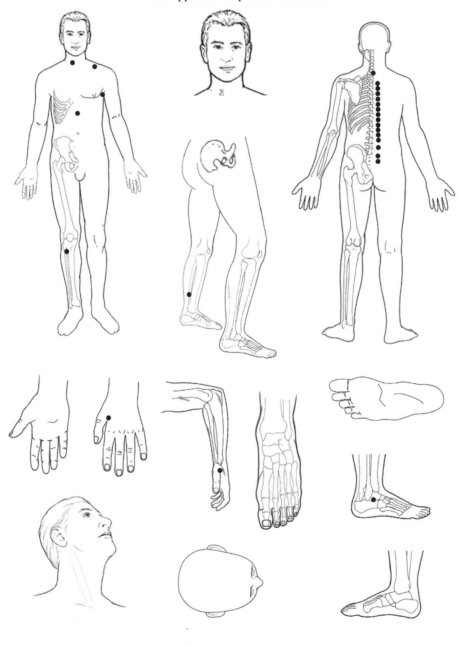

Food Poisoning -Detoxification

Emergency Nutritional Daily Menu	Maintenance Nutritional Daily Menu
Glyco: 9 tsp Phyto: 2 tsp Pre-Hormone: 3 tabs Essentials: 4 tabs	Glyco: 1/2 tsp Phyto: 1/2 tsp Pre-Hormone: 3 tabs Essentials: 4 tabs

see appendix for product definitions

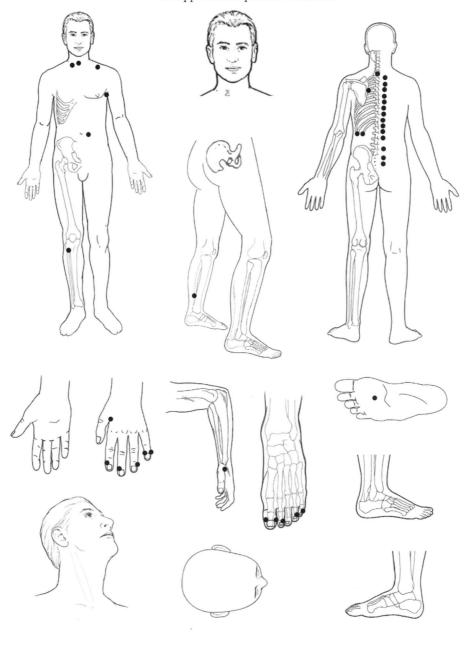

Fracture

Emergency Nutritional Daily Menu	Maintenance Nutritional Daily Menu
Glyco: 3 tsp Phyto: 1 tsp Pre-Hormone: 6 tabs Essentials: 4 tabs	Glyco: 1/2 tsp Phyto: 1/2 tsp Pre-Hormone: 3 tabs Essentials: 4 tabs

see appendix for product definitions

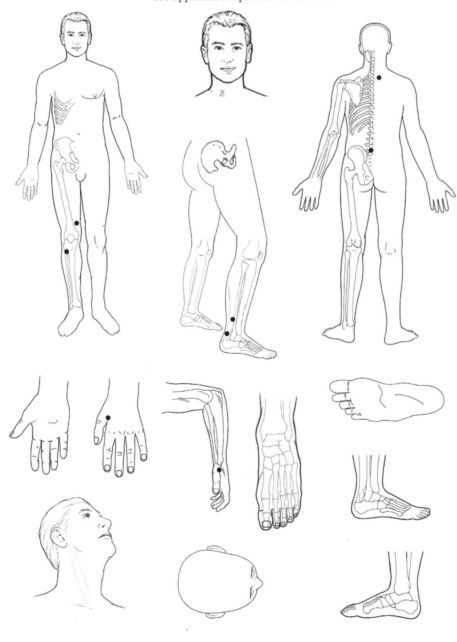

Frostbite

(stimulate meridian points surrounding injured area)

Emergency Nutritional Daily Menu	Maintenance Nutritional Daily Menu
Glyco: 6 tsp Phyto: 2 tsp Pre-Hormone: 6 tabs Essentials: 4 tabs	Glyco: 1 tsp Phyto: 1/2 tsp Pre-Hormone: 3 tabs Essentials: 4 tabs

see appendix for product definitions

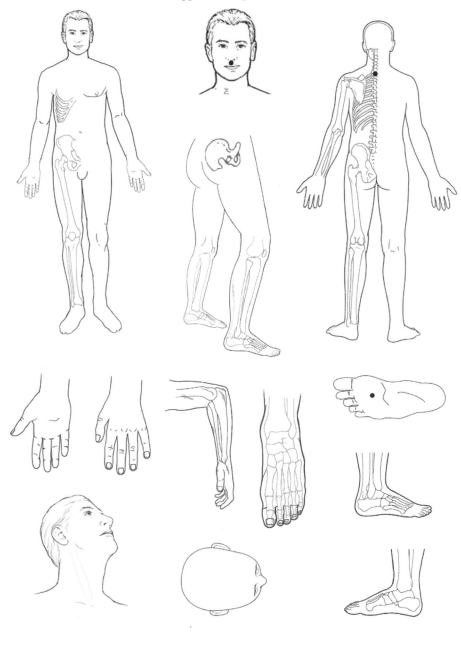

181

Fungal Infection

Emergency Nutritional Daily Menu	Maintenance Nutritional Daily Menu
Glyco: 6 tsp Phyto: 2 tsp Pre-Hormone: 6 tabs Cata-Blend: 4 tabs	Glyco: 1 tsp Phyto: 1/2 tsp Pre-Hormone: 3 tabs Cata-Blend: 4 tabs

see appendix for product definitions

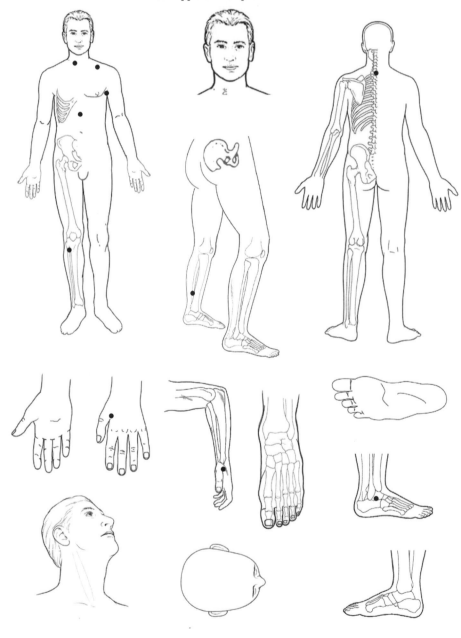

Furuncle/Carbuncle

Emergency Nutritional Daily Menu	Maintenance Nutritional Daily Menu
Glyco: 3 tsp Phyto: 2 tsp Pre-Hormone: 6 tabs Cata-Blend: 4 tabs	Glyco: 1 tsp Phyto: 1/2 tsp Pre-Hormone: 3 tabs Cata-Blend: 4 tabs

see appendix for product definitions

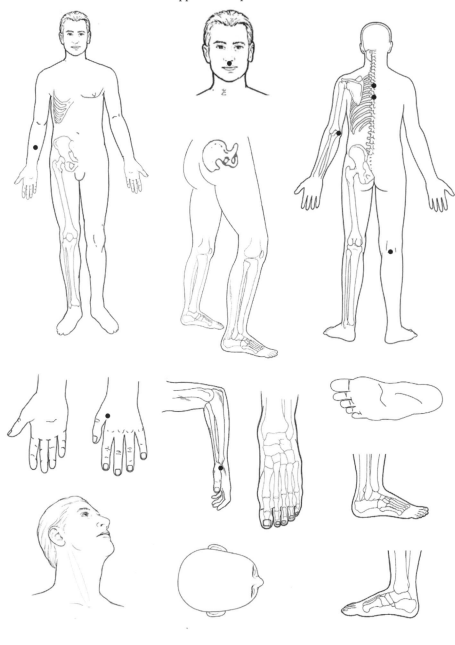

Gallbladder Dysfunction

Emergency Nutritional Daily Menu	Maintenance Nutritional Daily Menu
Glyco: 3 tsp Phyto: 2 tsp Pre-Hormone: 6 tabs Cata-Blend: 4 tabs	Glyco: 1 tsp Phyto: 1/2 tsp Pre-Hormone: 3 tabs Cata-Blend: 4 tabs

see appendix for product definitions

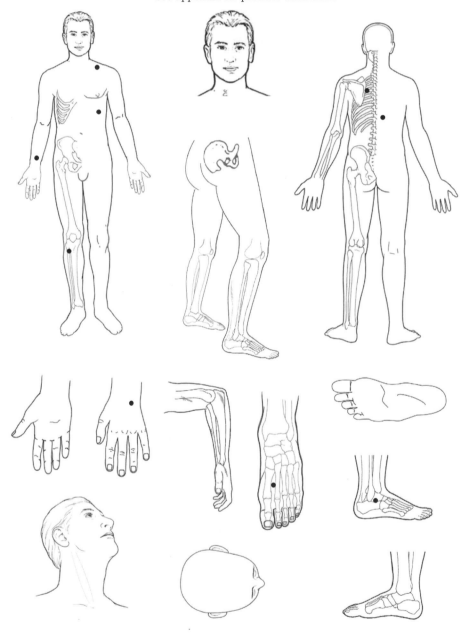

Gangrene

Emergency Nutritional Daily Menu	Maintenance Nutritional Daily Menu
Glyco: 6 tsp Phyto: 2 tsp Pre-Hormone: 6 tabs Cata-Blend: 6 tabs	Glyco: 2 tsp Phyto: 1 tsp Pre-Hormone: 3 tabs Cata-Blend: 4 tabs

see appendix for product definitions

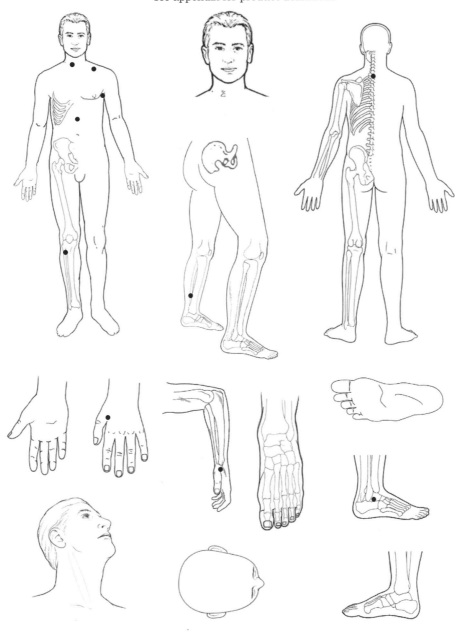

Gas (Intestinal)

Emergency Nutritional Daily Menu	Maintenance Nutritional Daily Menu
Glyco: 3 tsp Phyto: 1 tsp Pre-Hormone: 3 tabs Essentials: 4 tabs	Glyco: 1/2 tsp Phyto: 1/2 tsp Pre-Hormone: 3 tabs Essentials: 4 tabs

see appendix for product definitions

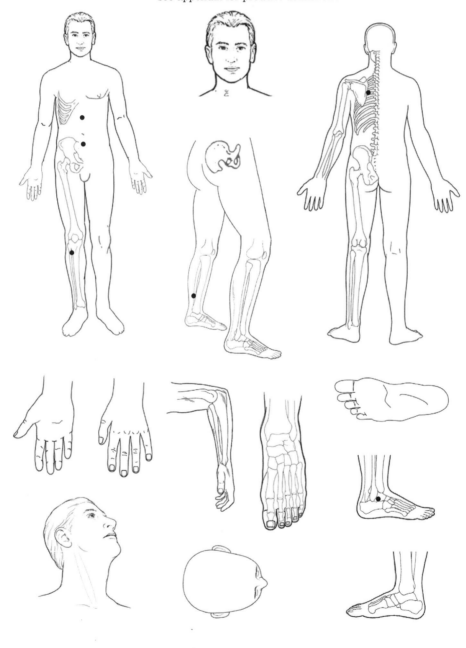

Gastric Ulcer

Emergency Nutritional Daily Menu	Maintenance Nutritional Daily Menu
Glyco: 3 tsp Phyto: 1 tsp Pre-Hormone: 3 tabs Essentials: 4 tabs	Glyco: 1 tsp Phyto: 1/2 tsp Pre-Hormone: 3 tabs Essentials: 4 tabs

see appendix for product definitions

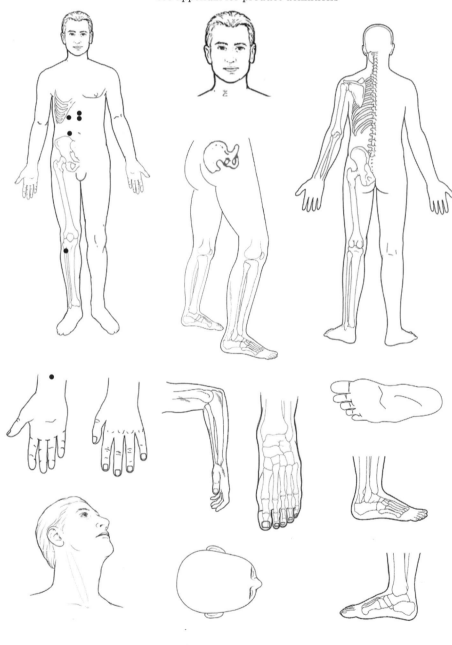

187

Gastroenteritis

Emergency Nutritional Daily Menu	Maintenance Nutritional Daily Menu
Glyco: 3 tsp Phyto: 1 tsp Pre-Hormone: 3 tabs Essentials: 4 tabs	Glyco: 1/2 tsp Phyto: 1/2 tsp Pre-Hormone: 3 tabs Essentials: 4 tabs

see appendix for product definitions

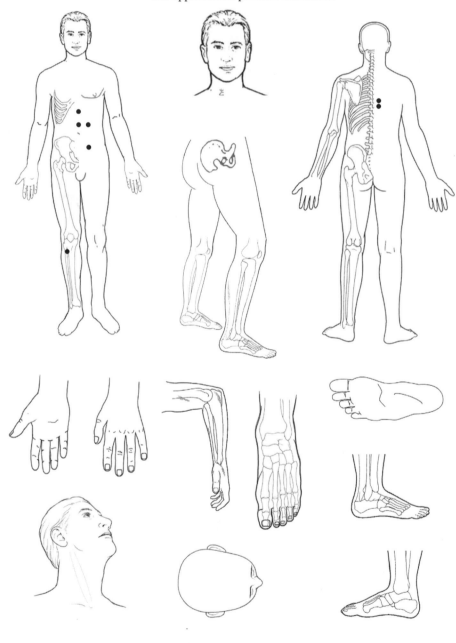

Gastroesophageal Reflux

Emergency Nutritional Daily Menu	Maintenance Nutritional Daily Menu
Glyco: 3 tsp Phyto: 1 tsp Pre-Hormone: 3 tabs Cata-Blend: 4 tabs	Glyco: 1 tsp Phyto: 1/2 tsp Pre-Hormone: 3 tabs Cata-Blend: 4 tabs

see appendix for product definitions

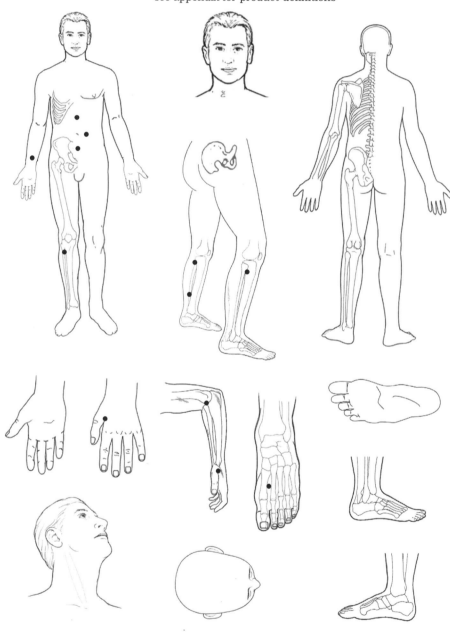

189

Gastroparesis

Emergency Nutritional Daily Menu	Maintenance Nutritional Daily Menu
Glyco: 3 tsp Phyto: 1 tsp Pre-Hormone: 3 tabs Cata-Blend: 4 tabs	Glyco: 1 tsp Phyto: 1/2 tsp Pre-Hormone: 3 tabs Cata-Blend: 4 tabs

see appendix for product definitions

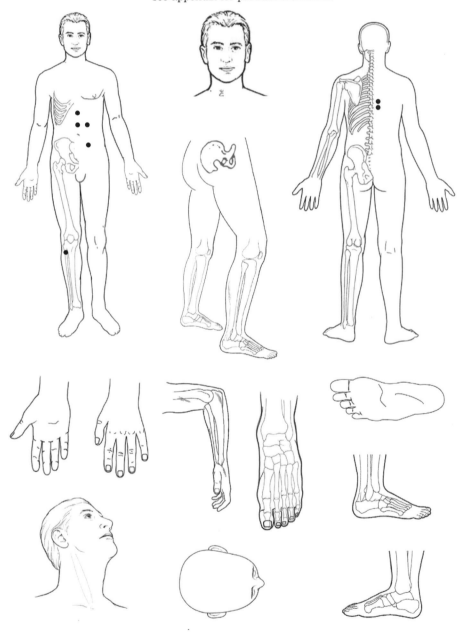

190

Genital Warts

Emergency Nutritional Daily Menu	Maintenance Nutritional Daily Menu
Glyco: 3 tsp Phyto: 2 tsp Pre-Hormone: 3 tabs Essentials: 4 tabs	Glyco: 1 tsp Phyto: 1/2 tsp Pre-Hormone: 3 tabs Essentials: 4 tabs

see appendix for product definitions

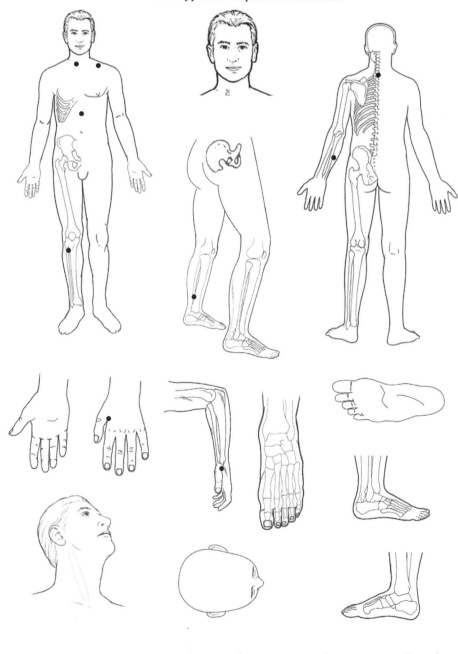

Gingivitis

Emergency Nutritional Daily Menu	Maintenance Nutritional Daily Menu
Glyco: 2 tsp Phyto: 1 tsp Pre-Hormone: 3 tabs Essentials: 4 tabs	Glyco: 1/2 tsp Phyto: 1/2 tsp Pre-Hormone: 3 tabs Essentials: 4 tabs

see appendix for product definitions

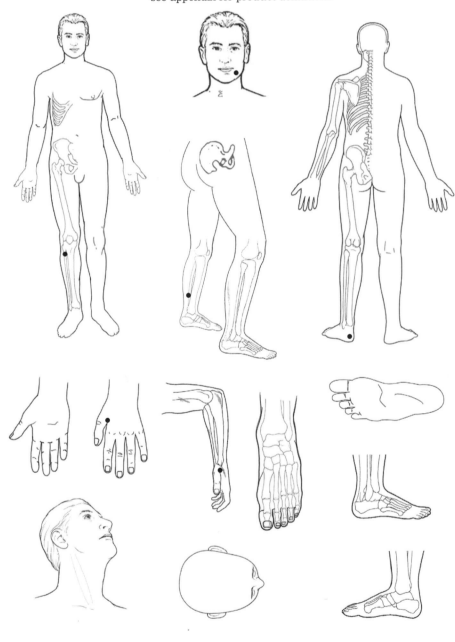

Glaucoma

Emergency Nutritional Daily Menu	Maintenance Nutritional Daily Menu
Glyco: 3 tsp Phyto: 2 tsp Pre-Hormone: 6 tabs Cata-Blend: 6 tabs	Glyco: 1 tsp Phyto: 1 tsp Pre-Hormone: 3 tabs Cata-Blend: 4 tabs

see appendix for product definitions

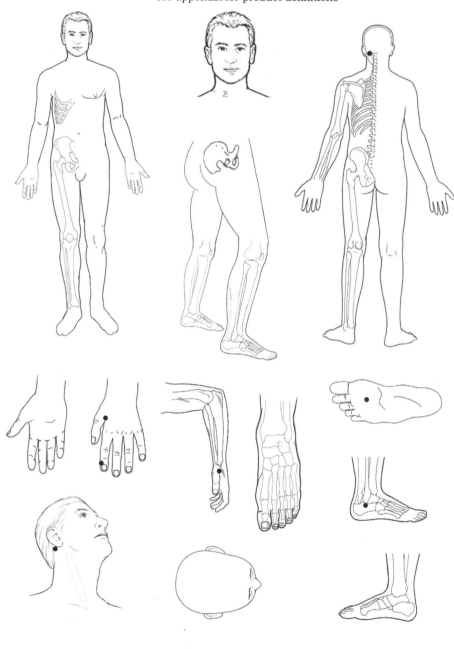

Glossitis

Emergency Nutritional Daily Menu	Maintenance Nutritional Daily Menu
Glyco: 2 tsp Phyto: 1 tsp Pre-Hormone: 3 tabs Essentials: 4 tabs	Glyco: 1 tsp Phyto: 1/2 tsp Pre-Hormone: 3 tabs Essentials: 4 tabs

see appendix for product definitions

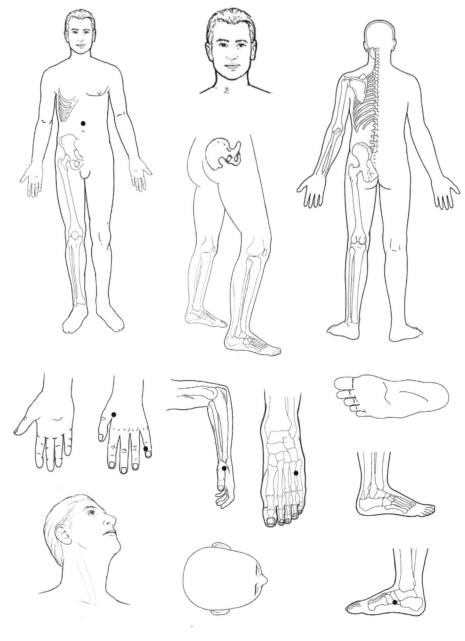

194

Glucose Intolerance

Emergency Nutritional Daily Menu	Maintenance Nutritional Daily Menu
Glyco: 3 tsp Phyto: 2 tsp Pre-Hormone: 4 tabs Cata-Blend: 4 tabs	Glyco: 1 tsp Phyto: 1 tsp Pre-Hormone: 4 tabs Cata-Blend: 4 tabs

see appendix for product definitions

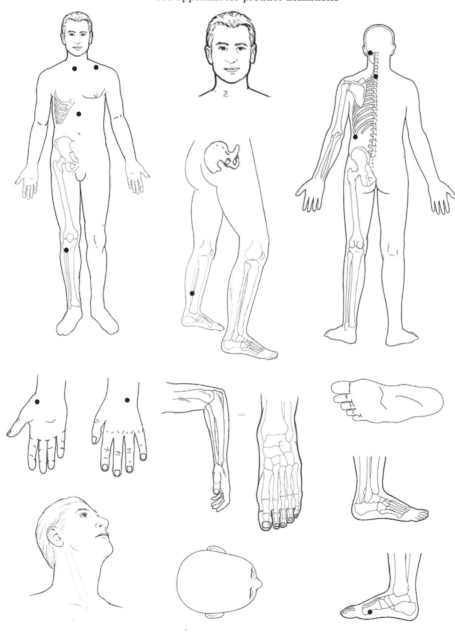

Goiter

Emergency Nutritional Daily Menu	Maintenance Nutritional Daily Menu
Glyco: 2 tsp Phyto: 1 tsp Pre-Hormone: 4 tabs Cata-Blend: 4 tabs	Glyco: 1 tsp Phyto: 1/2 tsp Pre-Hormone: 3 tabs Cata-Blend: 4 tabs

see appendix for product definitions

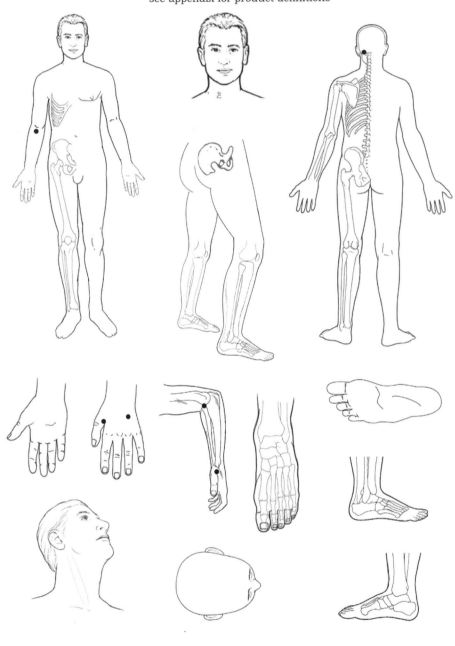

Gonorrhea

Emergency Nutritional Daily Menu	Maintenance Nutritional Daily Menu
Glyco: 3 tsp Phyto: 1 tsp Pre-Hormone: 3 tabs Essentials: 4 tabs	Glyco: 1 tsp Phyto: 1/2 tsp Pre-Hormone: 4 tabs Essentials: 4 tabs

see appendix for product definitions

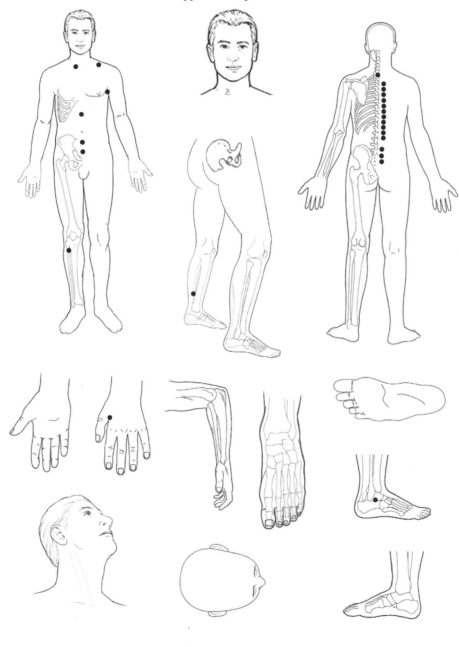

Gout

Emergency Nutritional Daily Menu	Maintenance Nutritional Daily Menu
Glyco: 3 tsp Phyto: 1 tsp Pre-Hormone: 6 tabs Cata-Blend: 6 tabs	Glyco: 1 tsp Phyto: 1/2 tsp Pre-Hormone: 3 tabs Cata-Blend: 4 tabs

see appendix for product definitions

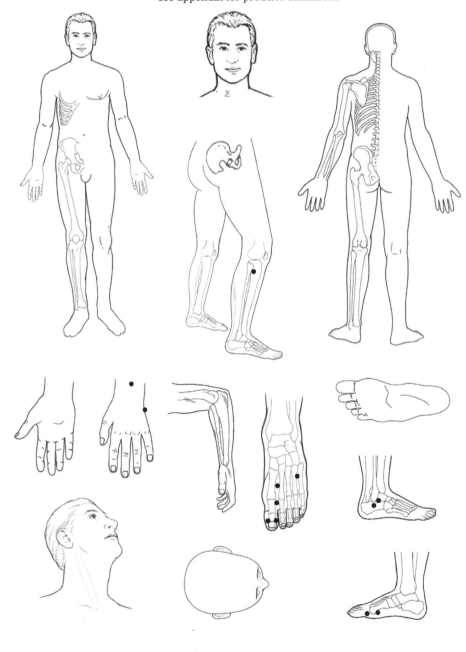

Graves' disease

Emergency Nutritional Daily Menu	Maintenance Nutritional Daily Menu
Glyco: 3 tsp Phyto: 1 tsp Pre-Hormone: 3 tabs Cata-Blend: 4 tabs	Glyco: 1 tsp Phyto: 1/2 tsp Pre-Hormone: 4 tabs Cata-Blend: 4 tabs

see appendix for product definitions

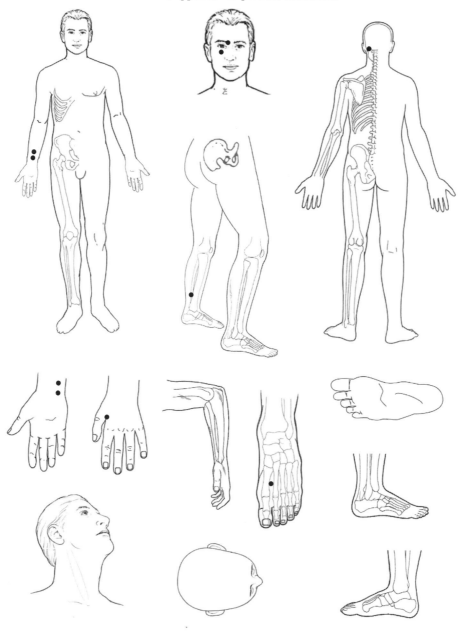

Hair Loss (Non-Genetic)

Emergency Nutritional Daily Menu	Maintenance Nutritional Daily Menu
Glyco: 2 tsp Phyto: 1 tsp Pre-Hormone: 6 tabs Essentials: 4 tabs	Glyco: 1 tsp Phyto: 1/2 tsp Pre-Hormone: 3 tabs Essentials: 4 tabs

see appendix for product definitions

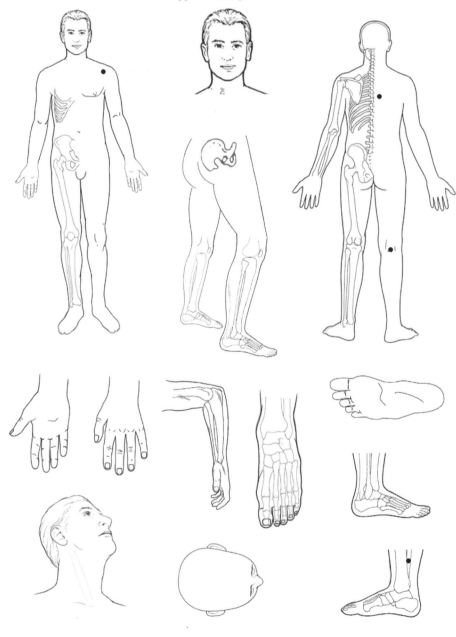

200

Hangover

Emergency Nutritional Daily Menu	Maintenance Nutritional Daily Menu
Glyco: 3 tsp Phyto: 2 tsp Pre-Hormone: 6 tabs Essentials: 4 tabs	Glyco: 1/2 tsp Phyto: 1/2 tsp Pre-Hormone: 3 tabs Essentials: 4 tabs

see appendix for product definitions

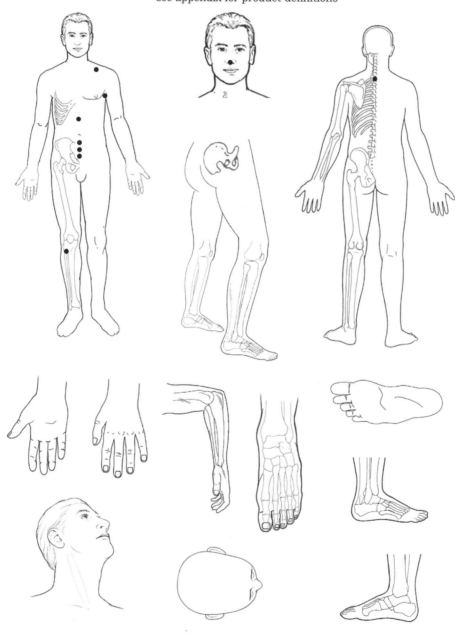

Hay Fever

Emergency Nutritional Daily Menu	Maintenance Nutritional Daily Menu
Glyco: 3 tsp Phyto: 1 tsp Pre-Hormone: 4 tabs Essentials: 4 tabs	Glyco: 1 tsp Phyto: 1/2 tsp Pre-Hormone: 3 tabs Essentials: 4 tabs

see appendix for product definitions

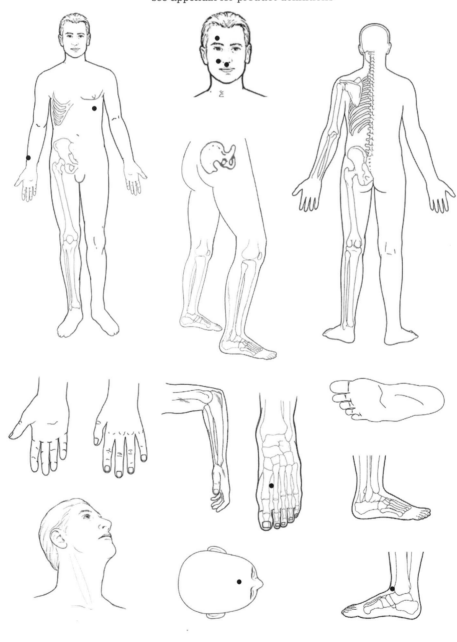

Headache

Emergency Nutritional Daily Menu	Maintenance Nutritional Daily Menu
Glyco: 3 tsp Phyto: 1 tsp Pre-Hormone: 6 tabs Essentials: 4 tabs	Glyco: 1 tsp Phyto: 1/2 tsp Pre-Hormone: 3 tabs Essentials: 4 tabs

see appendix for product definitions

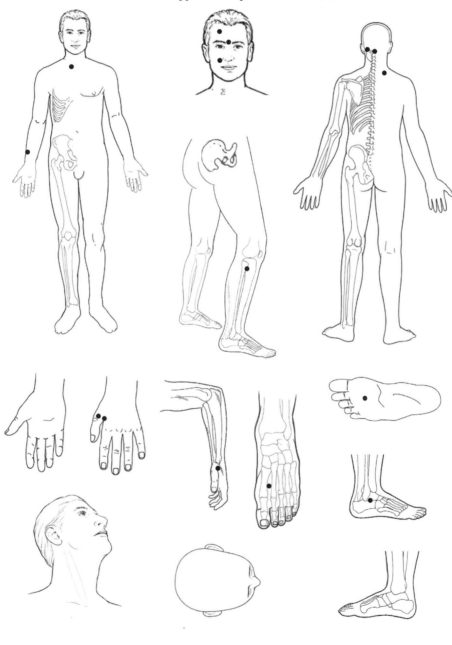

203

Hearing Loss

Emergency Nutritional Daily Menu	Maintenance Nutritional Daily Menu
Glyco: 6 tsp Phyto: 2 tsp Pre-Hormone: 4 tabs Essentials: 4 tabs	Glyco: 1 tsp Phyto: 1/2 tsp Pre-Hormone: 3 tabs Essentials: 4 tabs

see appendix for product definitions

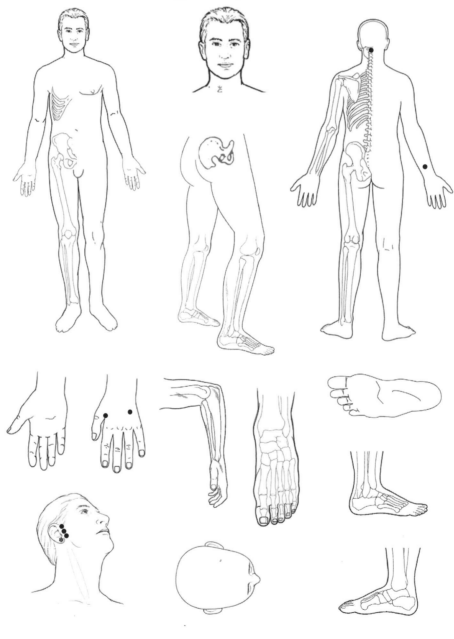

Heavy Metal Toxicity

Emergency Nutritional Daily Menu	Maintenance Nutritional Daily Menu
Glyco: 9 tsp Phyto: 3 tsp Pre-Hormone: 6 tabs Cata-Blend: 6 tabs	Glyco: 2 tsp Phyto: 1 tsp Pre-Hormone: 3 tabs Cata-Blend: 4 tabs

see appendix for product definitions

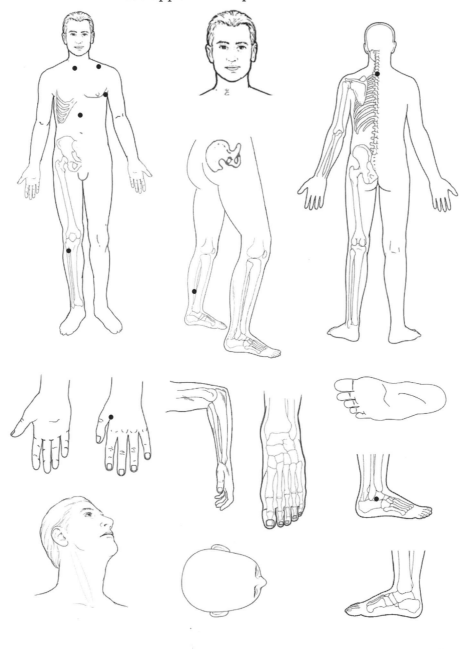

Hemiplegia Hemiparesis D/T Stroke

Emergency Nutritional Daily Menu	Maintenance Nutritional Daily Menu
Glyco: 9 tsp Phyto: 2 tsp Pre-Hormone: 6 tabs Cata-Blend: 6 tabs	Glyco: 2 tsp Phyto: 1 tsp Pre-Hormone: 4 tabs Cata-Blend: 4 tabs

see appendix for product definitions

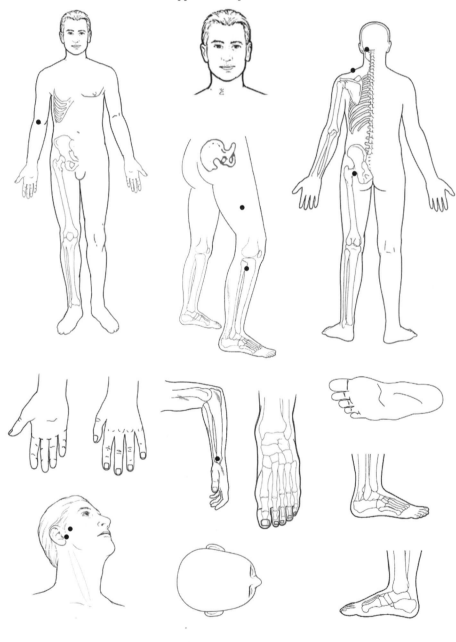

Hepatitis A

Emergency Nutritional Daily Menu	Maintenance Nutritional Daily Menu
Glyco: 9 tsp Phyto: 2 tsp Pre-Hormone: 4 tabs Cata-Blend: 4 tabs	Glyco: 1/2 tsp Phyto: 1/2 tsp Pre-Hormone: 4 tabs Cata-Blend: 4 tabs

see appendix for product definitions

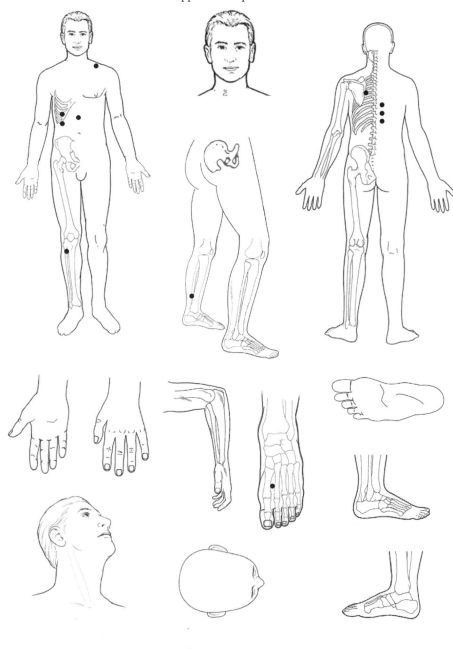

Hepatitis B

Emergency Nutritional Daily Menu	Maintenance Nutritional Daily Menu
Glyco: 9 tsp Phyto: 2 tsp Pre-Hormone: 4 tabs Cata-Blend: 4 tabs	Glyco: 2 tsp Phyto: 1 tsp Pre-Hormone: 4 tabs Cata-Blend: 4 tabs

see appendix for product definitions

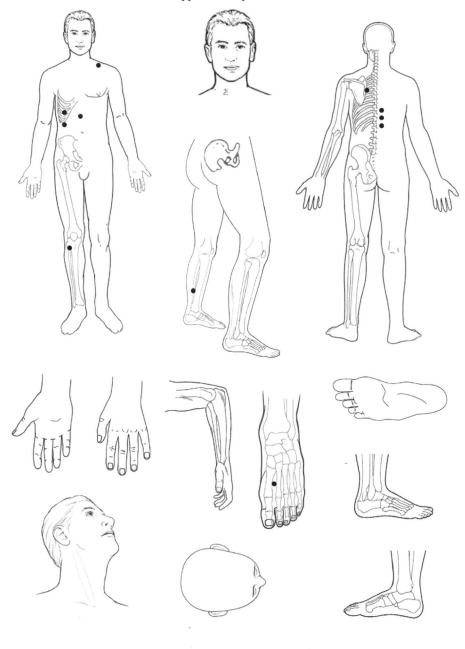

Hepatitis C, Chronic

Emergency Nutritional Daily Menu	Maintenance Nutritional Daily Menu
Glyco: 9 tsp Phyto: 2 tsp Pre-Hormone: 4 tabs Cata-Blend: 6 tabs	Glyco: 2 tsp Phyto: 1 tsp Pre-Hormone: 4 tabs Cata-Blend: 4 tabs

see appendix for product definitions

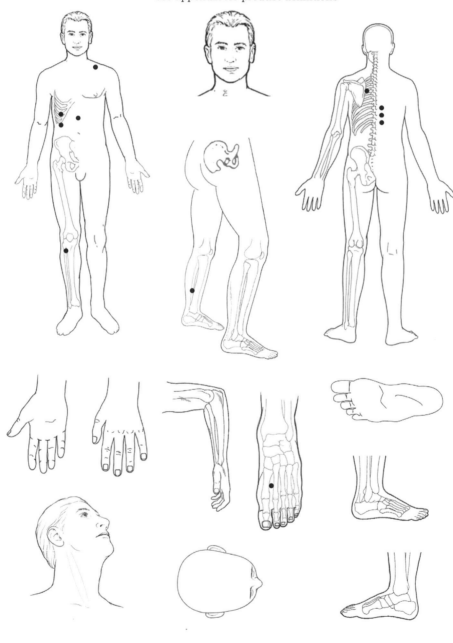

Herniated Intervertebral Disc
(stimulate points surrounding areas of pain)

Emergency Nutritional Daily Menu	Maintenance Nutritional Daily Menu
Glyco: 6 tsp Phyto: 1 tsp Pre-Hormone: 6 tabs Cata-Blend: 4 tabs	Glyco: 2 tsp Phyto: 1 tsp Pre-Hormone: 4 tabs Cata-Blend: 4 tabs

see appendix for product definitions

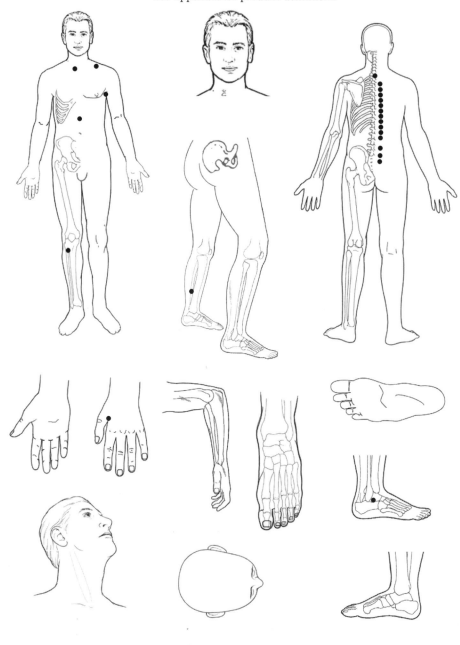

Herpes Simplex
(apply soft laser on affected area)

Emergency Nutritional Daily Menu	Maintenance Nutritional Daily Menu
Glyco: 3 tsp Phyto: 1 tsp Pre-Hormone: 6 tabs Cata-Blend: 4 tabs	Glyco: 1 tsp Phyto: 1 tsp Pre-Hormone: 3 tabs Cata-Blend: 4 tabs

see appendix for product definitions

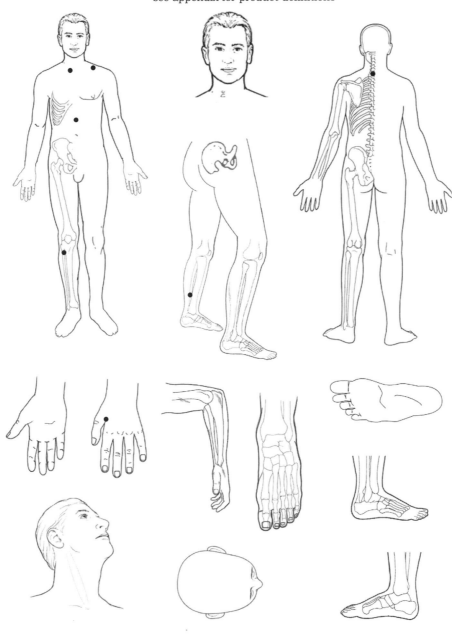

211

Herpes Zoster

Emergency Nutritional Daily Menu	Maintenance Nutritional Daily Menu
Glyco: 6 tsp Phyto: 1 tsp Pre-Hormone: 6 tabs Cata-Blend: 4 tabs	Glyco: 1 tsp Phyto: 1 tsp Pre-Hormone: 3 tabs Cata-Blend: 4 tabs

see appendix for product definitions

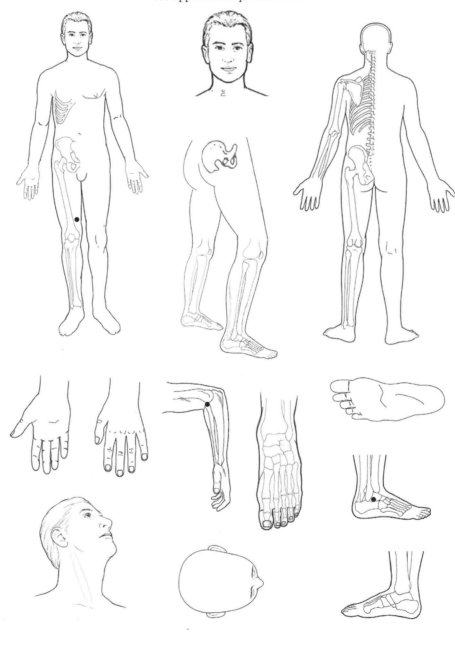

Herpes, Genital

(apply soft laser on affected area)

Emergency Nutritional Daily Menu	Maintenance Nutritional Daily Menu
Glyco: 3 tsp Phyto: 1 tsp Pre-Hormone: 6 tabs Cata-Blend: 4 tabs	Glyco: 1 tsp Phyto: 1 tsp Pre-Hormone: 3 tabs Cata-Blend: 4 tabs

see appendix for product definitions

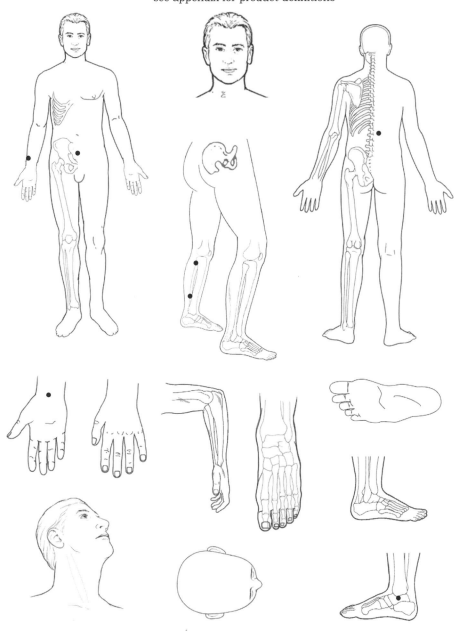

213

HIV Disease

Emergency Nutritional Daily Menu	Maintenance Nutritional Daily Menu
Glyco: 12 tsp Phyto: 3 tsp Pre-Hormone: 6 tabs Cata-Blend: 6 tabs	Glyco: 3 tsp Phyto: 2 tsp Pre-Hormone: 4 tabs Cata-Blend: 4 tabs

see appendix for product definitions

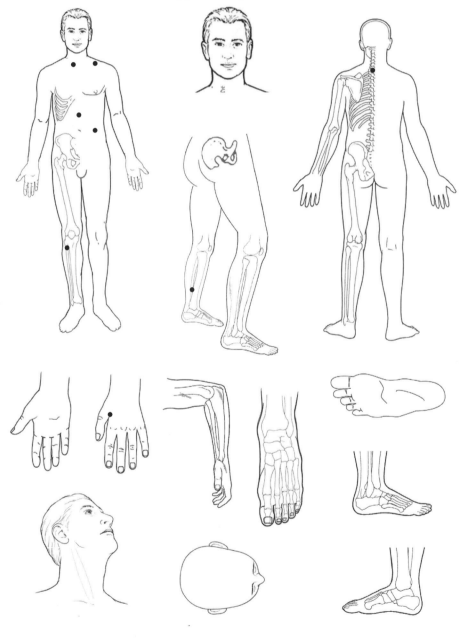

Hives

Emergency Nutritional Daily Menu	Maintenance Nutritional Daily Menu
Glyco: 6 tsp Phyto: 2 tsp Pre-Hormone: 4 tabs Essentials: 4 tabs	Glyco: 1/2 tsp Phyto: 1/2 tsp Pre-Hormone: 3 tabs Essentials: 4 tabs

see appendix for product definitions

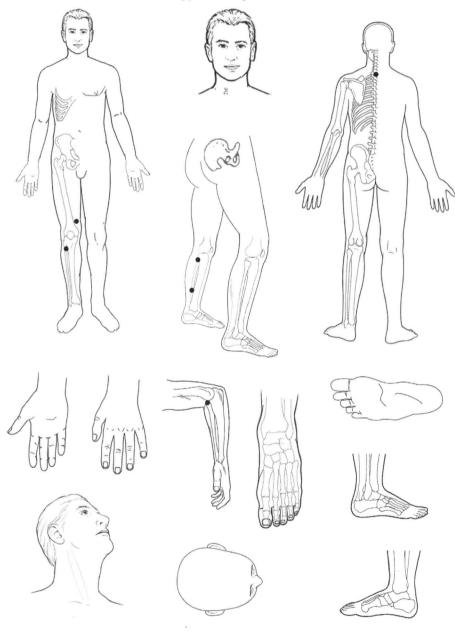

215

Hodgkins Disease

Emergency Nutritional Daily Menu	Maintenance Nutritional Daily Menu
Glyco: 12 tsp Phyto: 3 tsp Pre-Hormone: 6 tabs Cata-Blend: 6 tabs	Glyco: 3 tsp Phyto: 2 tsp Pre-Hormone: 4 tabs Cata-Blend: 6 tabs

see appendix for product definitions

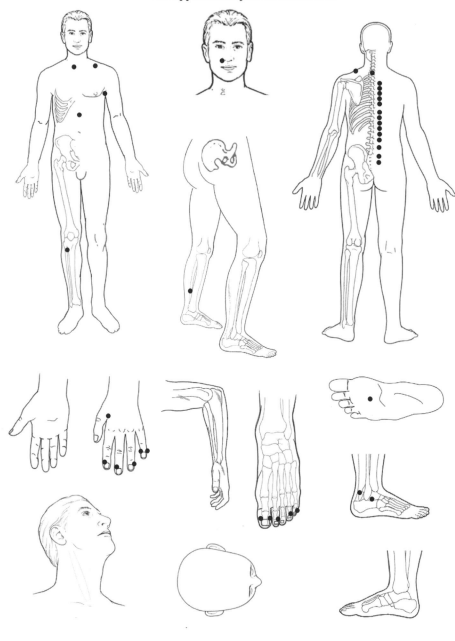

Hyperaldosteronism

Emergency Nutritional Daily Menu	Maintenance Nutritional Daily Menu
Glyco: 3 tsp Phyto: 2 tsp Pre-Hormone: 6 tabs Essentials: 4 tabs	Glyco: 2 tsp Phyto: 1 tsp Pre-Hormone: 4 tabs Essentials: 4 tabs

see appendix for product definitions

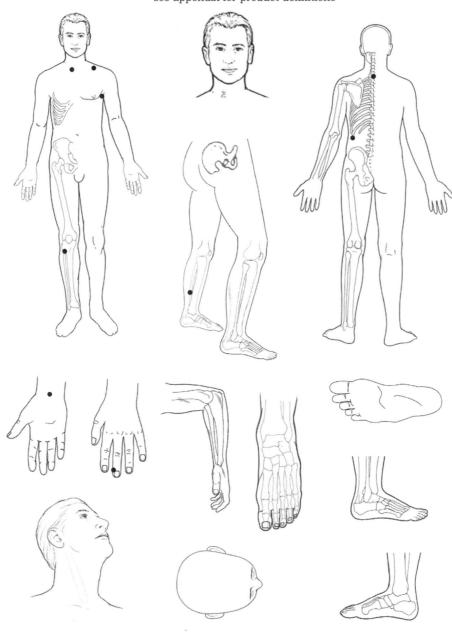

Hypercholesterolemia

Emergency Nutritional Daily Menu	Maintenance Nutritional Daily Menu
Glyco: 2 tsp Phyto: 2 tsp Pre-Hormone: 6 tabs Cata-Blend: 4 tabs	Glyco: 2 tsp Phyto: 1 tsp Pre-Hormone: 4 tabs Cata-Blend: 4 tabs

see appendix for product definitions

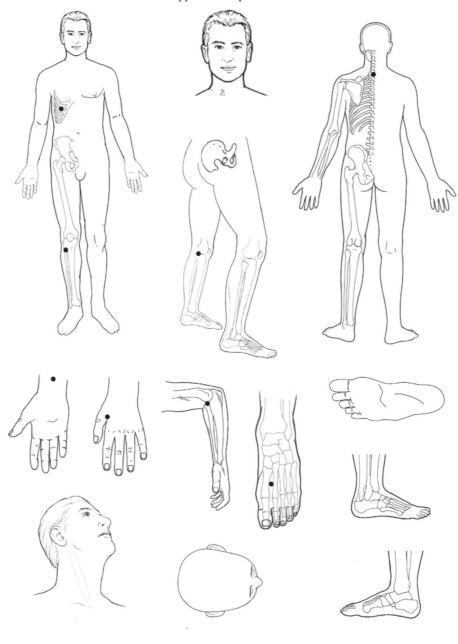

Hyperesthesia

Emergency Nutritional Daily Menu	Maintenance Nutritional Daily Menu
Glyco: 9 tsp Phyto: 1 tsp Pre-Hormone: 6 tabs Cata-Blend: 4 tabs	Glyco: 2 tsp Phyto: 1 tsp Pre-Hormone: 3 tabs Cata-Blend: 4 tabs

see appendix for product definitions

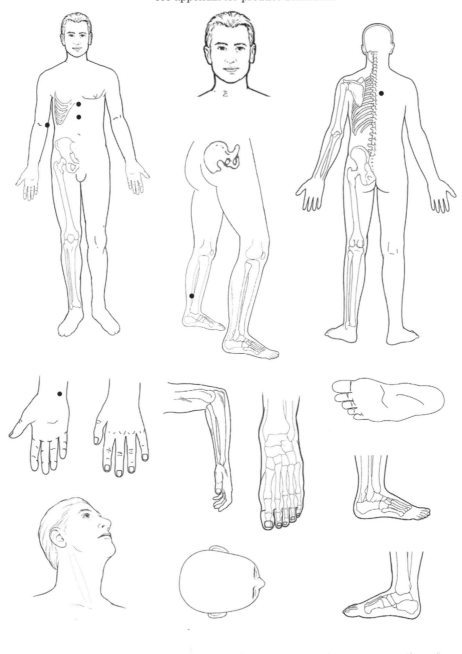

Hyperhidrosos

Emergency Nutritional Daily Menu	Maintenance Nutritional Daily Menu
Glyco: 6 tsp Phyto: 2 tsp Pre-Hormone: 6 tabs Cata-Blend: 4 tabs	Glyco: 2 tsp Phyto: 1/2 tsp Pre-Hormone: 3 tabs Cata-Blend: 4 tabs

see appendix for product definitions

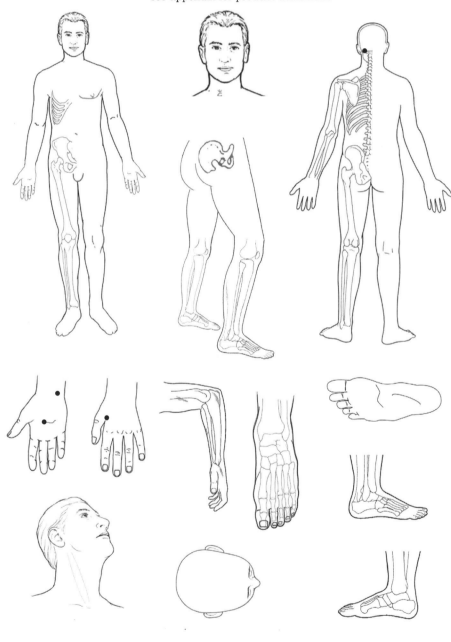

220

Hyperlipidemia (Triglycerides)

Emergency Nutritional Daily Menu	Maintenance Nutritional Daily Menu
Glyco: 6 tsp Phyto: 2 tsp Pre-Hormone: 6 tabs Cata-Blend: 4 tabs	Glyco: 2 tsp Phyto: 1/2 tsp Pre-Hormone: 3 tabs Cata-Blend: 4 tabs

see appendix for product definitions

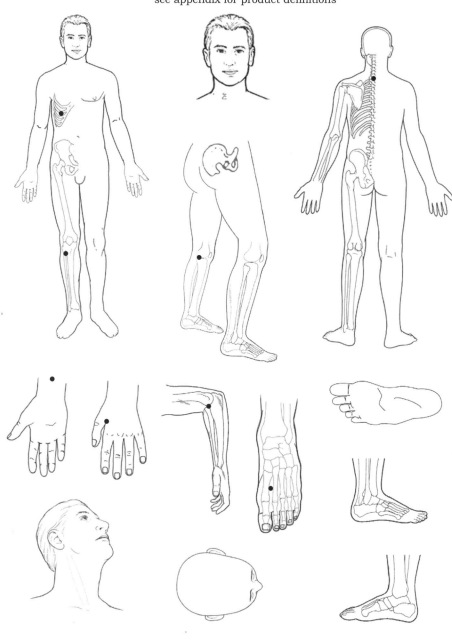

Hypertension

Emergency Nutritional Daily Menu	Maintenance Nutritional Daily Menu
Glyco: 6 tsp Phyto: 2 tsp Pre-Hormone: 6 tabs Cata-Blend: 4 tabs	Glyco: 2 tsp Phyto: 1 tsp Pre-Hormone: 3 tabs Cata-Blend: 4 tabs

see appendix for product definitions

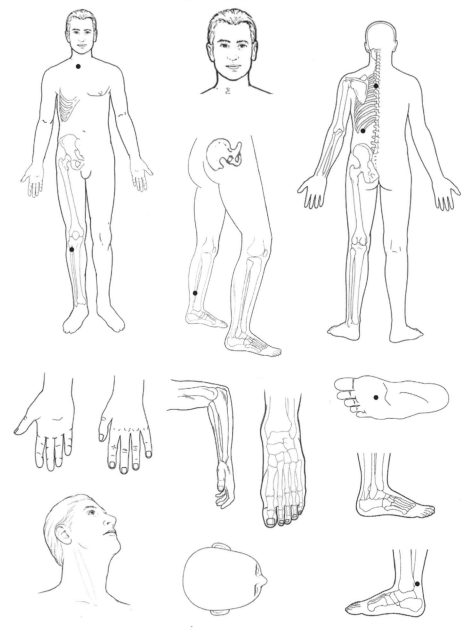

Hyperthyroidism

Emergency Nutritional Daily Menu	Maintenance Nutritional Daily Menu
Glyco: 6 tsp Phyto: 1 tsp Pre-Hormone: 3 tabs Cata-Blend: 4 tabs	Glyco: 1 tsp Phyto: 1/2 tsp Pre-Hormone: 3 tabs Cata-Blend: 4 tabs

see appendix for product definitions

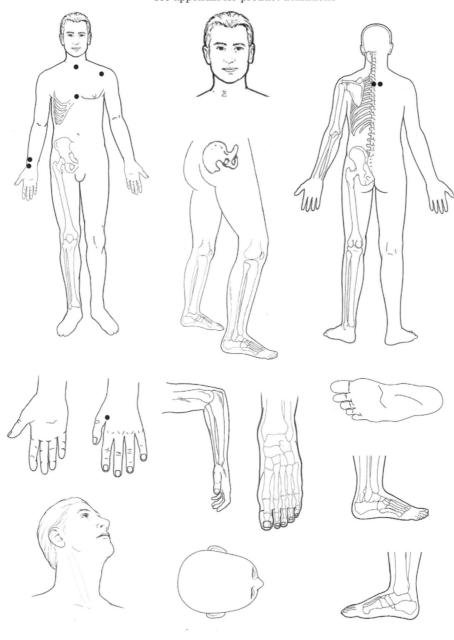

Hyperventilation

Emergency Nutritional Daily Menu	Maintenance Nutritional Daily Menu
Glyco: 3 tsp Phyto: 1/2 tsp Pre-Hormone: 4 tabs Essentials: 4 tabs	Glyco: 1/2 tsp Phyto: 1/2 tsp Pre-Hormone: 3 tabs Essentials: 4 tabs

see appendix for product definitions

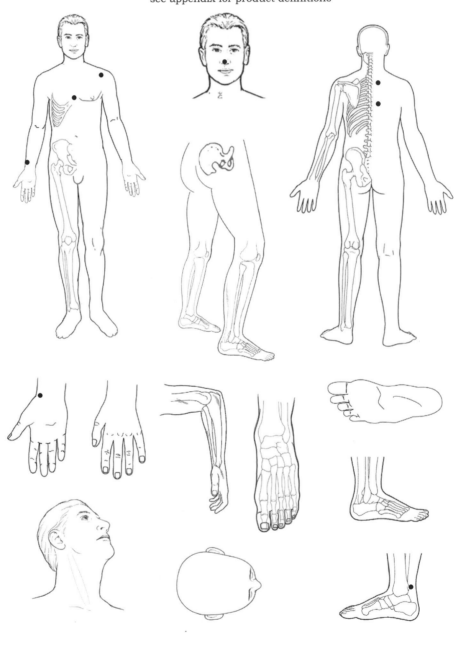

Hypoglycemia

Emergency Nutritional Daily Menu	Maintenance Nutritional Daily Menu
Glyco: 6 tsp Phyto: 1 tsp Pre-Hormone: 6 tabs Cata-Blend: 4 tabs	Glyco: 1 tsp Phyto: 1/2 tsp Pre-Hormone: 3 tabs Cata-Blend: 4 tabs

see appendix for product definitions

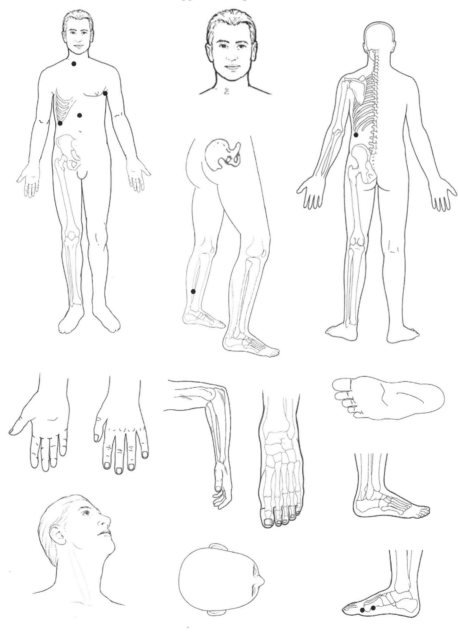

Hysterectomy

Emergency Nutritional Daily Menu	Maintenance Nutritional Daily Menu
Glyco: 6 tsp Phyto: 2 tsp Pre-Hormone: 6 tabs Essentials: 4 tabs	Glyco: 1 tsp Phyto: 1/2 tsp Pre-Hormone: 3 tabs Essentials: 4 tabs

see appendix for product definitions

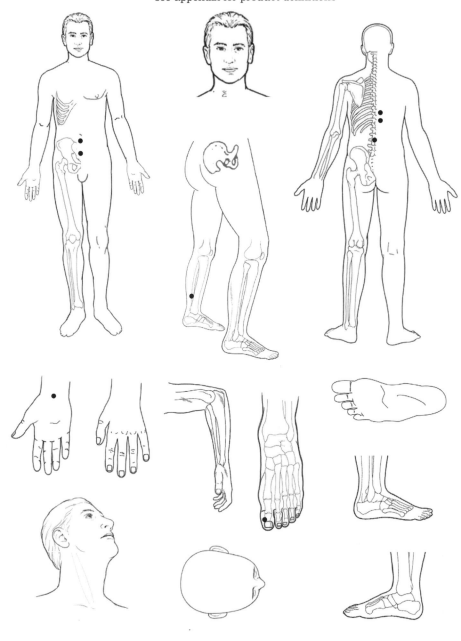

226

Ileitis

Emergency Nutritional Daily Menu	Maintenance Nutritional Daily Menu
Glyco: 9 tsp Phyto: 2 tsp Pre-Hormone: 4 tabs Cata-Blend: 4 tabs	Glyco: 2 tsp Phyto: 1 tsp Pre-Hormone: 3 tabs Cata-Blend: 4 tabs

see appendix for product definitions

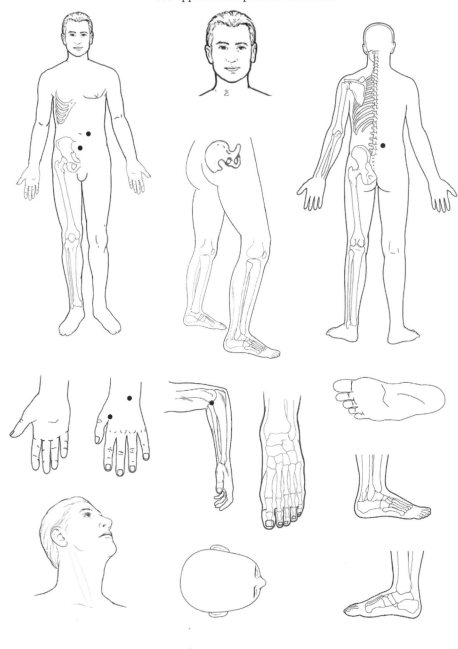

227

Immune Deficiency (Chronic)

Emergency Nutritional Daily Menu	Maintenance Nutritional Daily Menu
Glyco: 9 tsp Phyto: 2 tsp Pre-Hormone: 4 tabs Cata-Blend: 6 tabs	Glyco: 3 tsp Phyto: 2 tsp Pre-Hormone: 3 tabs Cata-Blend: 6 tabs

see appendix for product definitions

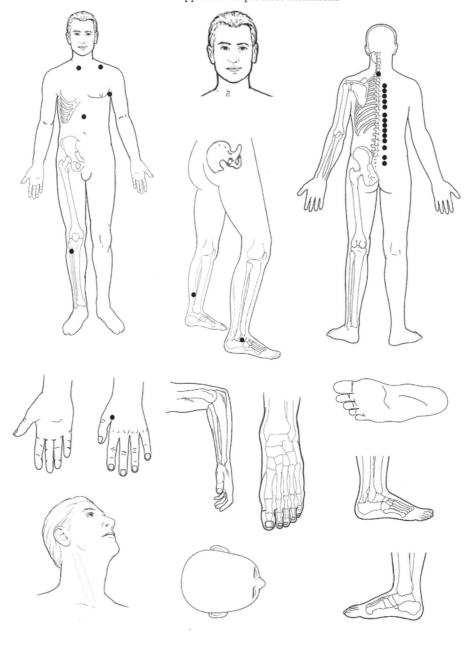

Immune System Support

Emergency Nutritional Daily Menu	Maintenance Nutritional Daily Menu
Glyco: 6 tsp Phyto: 1 tsp Pre-Hormone: 4 tabs Cata-Blend: 4 tabs	Glyco: 2 tsp Phyto: 1 tsp Pre-Hormone: 3 tabs Cata-Blend: 4 tabs

see appendix for product definitions

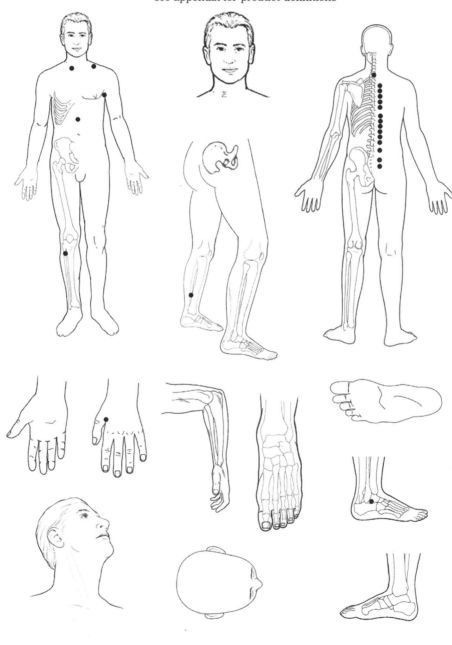

Impetigo

Emergency Nutritional Daily Menu	Maintenance Nutritional Daily Menu
Glyco: 3 tsp Phyto: 1 tsp Pre-Hormone: 3 tabs Cata-Blend: 4 tabs	Glyco: 1 tsp Phyto: 1/2 tsp Pre-Hormone: 3 tabs Cata-Blend: 4 tabs

see appendix for product definitions

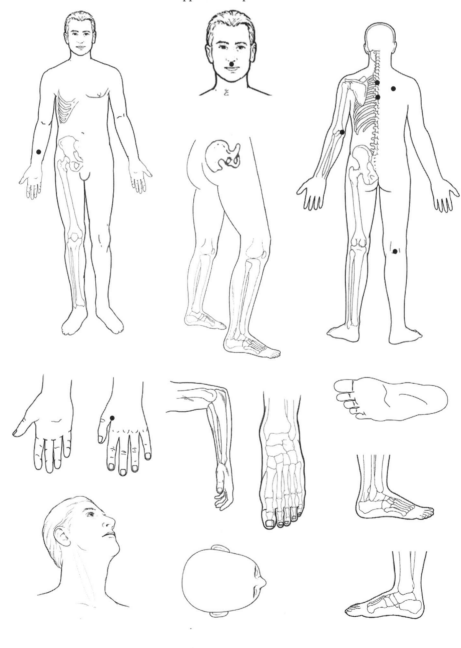

Impotence (Organic Erectile Dysfunction)

Emergency Nutritional Daily Menu	Maintenance Nutritional Daily Menu
Glyco: 3 tsp Phyto: 2 tsp Pre-Hormone: 6 tabs Cata-Blend: 4 tabs	Glyco: 2 tsp Phyto: 1 tsp Pre-Hormone: 4 tabs Cata-Blend: 4 tabs

see appendix for product definitions

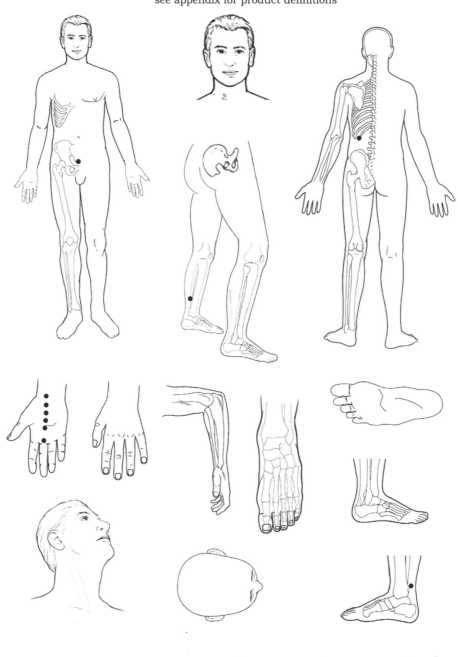

231

Incontinence Enuresis

Emergency Nutritional Daily Menu	Maintenance Nutritional Daily Menu
Glyco: 3 tsp Phyto: 1 tsp Pre-Hormone: 4 tabs Cata-Blend: 4 tabs	Glyco: 1 tsp Phyto: 1/2 tsp Pre-Hormone: 3 tabs Cata-Blend: 4 tabs

see appendix for product definitions

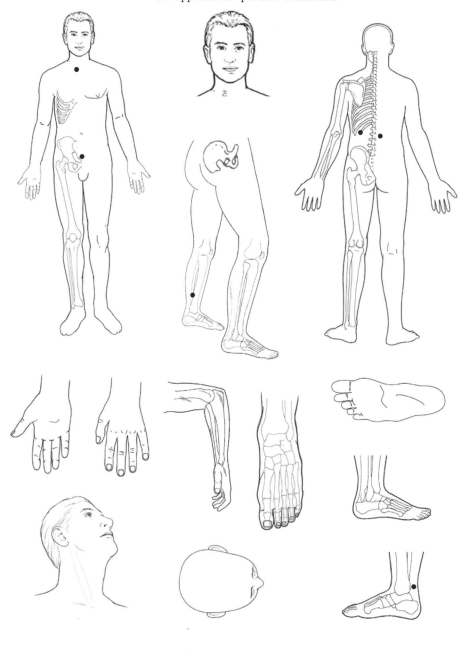

Infection (Systemic)

Emergency Nutritional Daily Menu	Maintenance Nutritional Daily Menu
Glyco: 12 tsp Phyto: 2 tsp Pre-Hormone: 6 tabs Cata-Blend: 6 tabs	Glyco: 2 tsp Phyto: 1 tsp Pre-Hormone: 3 tabs Cata-Blend: 4 tabs

see appendix for product definitions

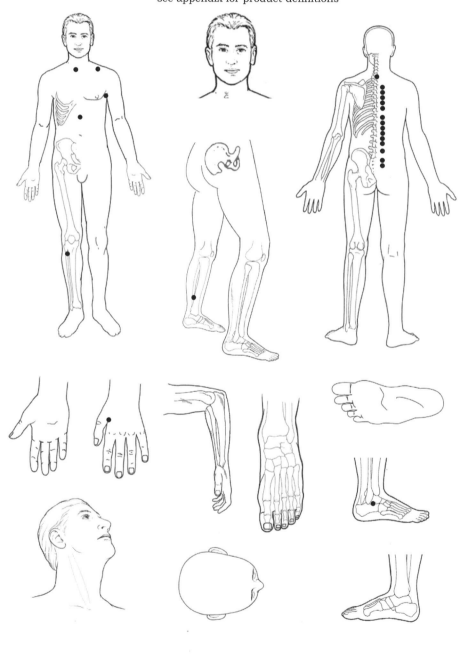

233

Infertility (Female)

Emergency Nutritional Daily Menu	Maintenance Nutritional Daily Menu
Glyco: 3 tsp Phyto: 2 tsp Pre-Hormone: 6 tabs Cata-Blend: 4 tabs	Glyco: 2 tsp Phyto: 1 tsp Pre-Hormone: 3 tabs Cata-Blend: 4 tabs

see appendix for product definitions

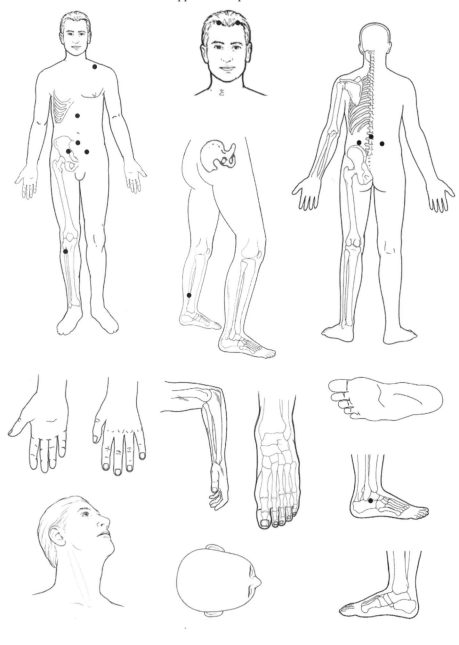

Infertility (Male)

Emergency Nutritional Daily Menu	Maintenance Nutritional Daily Menu
Glyco: 3 tsp Phyto: 2 tsp Pre-Hormone: 6 tabs Cata-Blend: 4 tabs	Glyco: 2 tsp Phyto: 1 tsp Pre-Hormone: 3 tabs Cata-Blend: 4 tabs

see appendix for product definitions

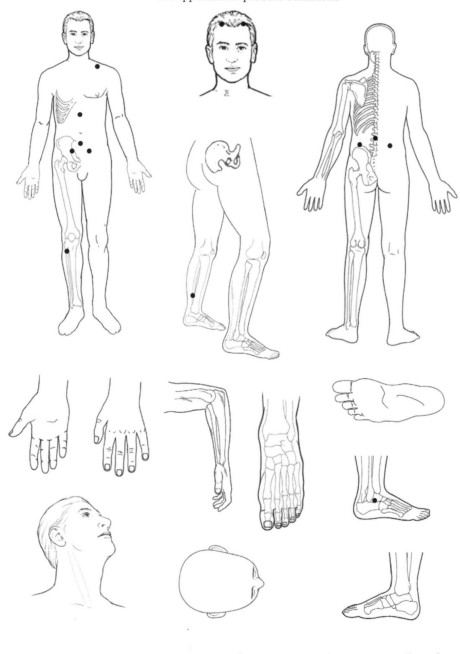

235

Inflammation (Systemic)

Emergency Nutritional Daily Menu	Maintenance Nutritional Daily Menu
Glyco: 12 tsp Phyto: 2 tsp Pre-Hormone: 6 tabs Cata-Blend: 6 tabs	Glyco: 2 tsp Phyto: 1 tsp Pre-Hormone: 3 tabs Cata-Blend: 4 tabs

see appendix for product definitions

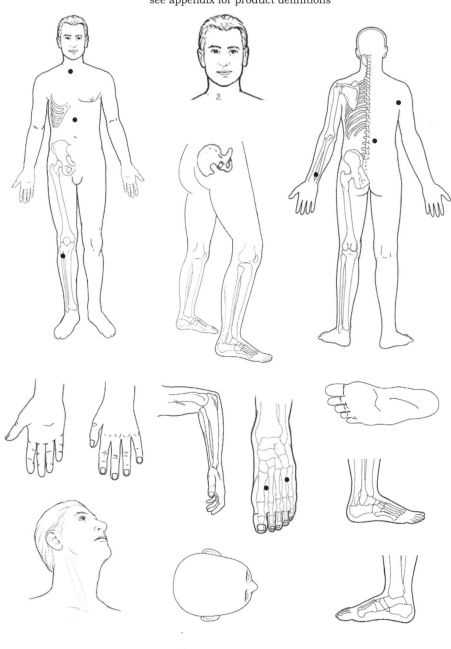

236

Influenza w/ Respiratory Manifestations

Emergency Nutritional Daily Menu	Maintenance Nutritional Daily Menu
Glyco: 6 tsp Phyto: 2 tsp Pre-Hormone: 6 tabs Cata-Blend: 4 tabs	Glyco: 1 tsp Phyto: 1 tsp Pre-Hormone: 3 tabs Cata-Blend: 4 tabs

see appendix for product definitions

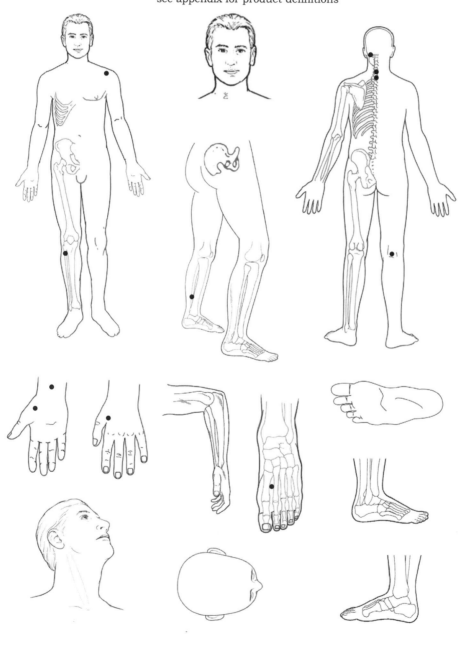

237

Insect Bite (venomous)

Emergency Nutritional Daily Menu	Maintenance Nutritional Daily Menu
Glyco: 12 tsp Phyto: 2 tsp Pre-Hormone: 6 tabs Essentials: 4 tabs	Glyco: 1/2 tsp Phyto: 1/2 tsp Pre-Hormone: 3 tabs Essentials: 4 tabs

see appendix for product definitions

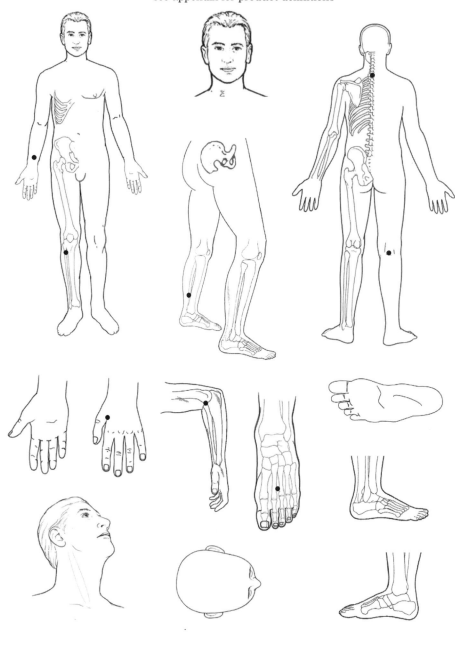

Insomnia

Emergency Nutritional Daily Menu	Maintenance Nutritional Daily Menu
Glyco: 3 tsp Phyto: 1 tsp Pre-Hormone: 4 tabs Essentials: 4 tabs	Glyco: 1 tsp Phyto: 1/2 tsp Pre-Hormone: 3 tabs Essentials: 4 tabs

see appendix for product definitions

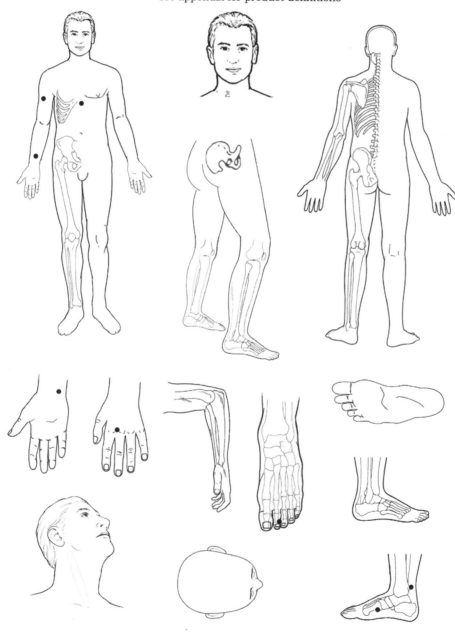

Intestinal Malabsorption

Emergency Nutritional Daily Menu	Maintenance Nutritional Daily Menu
Glyco: 3 tsp Phyto: 1 tsp Pre-Hormone: 6 tabs Essentials: 4 tabs	Glyco: 1 tsp Phyto: 1 tsp Pre-Hormone: 3 tabs Essentials: 4 tabs

see appendix for product definitions

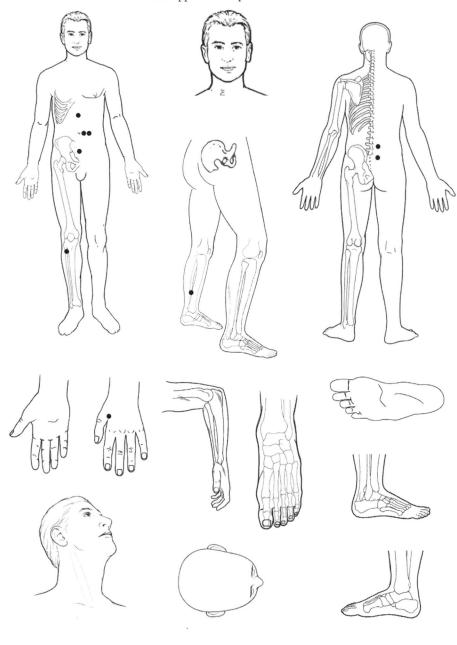

Irritable Bowel Syndrome (IBS)

Emergency Nutritional Daily Menu	Maintenance Nutritional Daily Menu
Glyco: 3 tsp Phyto: 1 tsp Pre-Hormone: 6 tabs Cata-Blend: 4 tabs	Glyco: 1 tsp Phyto: 1/2 tsp Pre-Hormone: 3 tabs Cata-Blend: 4 tabs

see appendix for product definitions

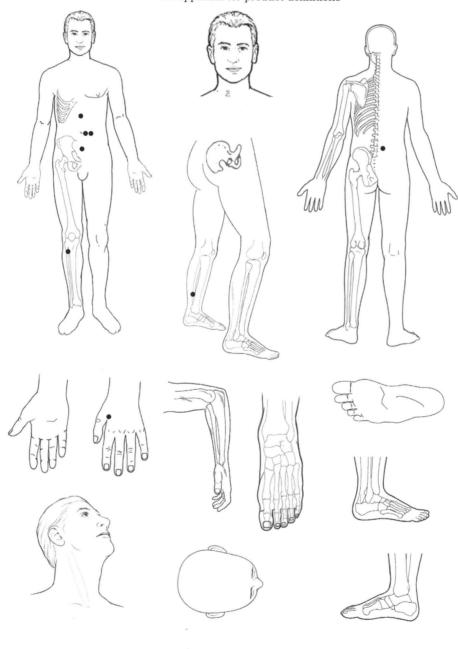

© 2003 Schlachter & Aristotle   241

Ischemic Bowel Disease

Emergency Nutritional Daily Menu	Maintenance Nutritional Daily Menu
Glyco: 9 tsp Phyto: 2 tsp Pre-Hormone: 6 tabs Cata-Blend: 6 tabs	Glyco: 1 tsp Phyto: 1/2 tsp Pre-Hormone: 3 tabs Cata-Blend: 4 tabs

see appendix for product definitions

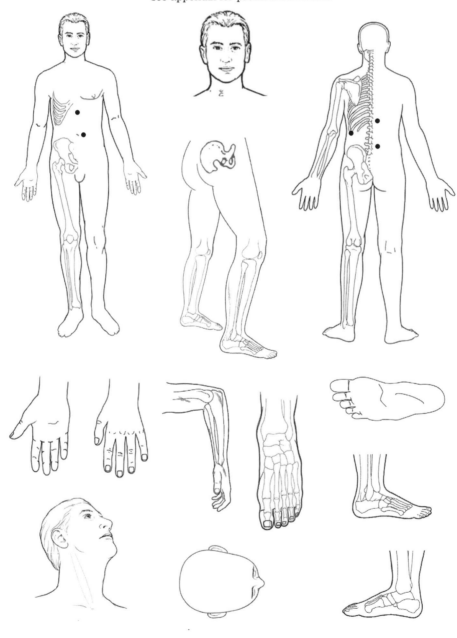

Itching (Pruritis)

Emergency Nutritional Daily Menu	Maintenance Nutritional Daily Menu
Glyco: 4 tsp Phyto: 2 tsp Pre-Hormone: 6 tabs Essentials: 4 tabs	Glyco: 2 tsp Phyto: 1 tsp Pre-Hormone: 3 tabs Essentials: 4 tabs

see appendix for product definitions

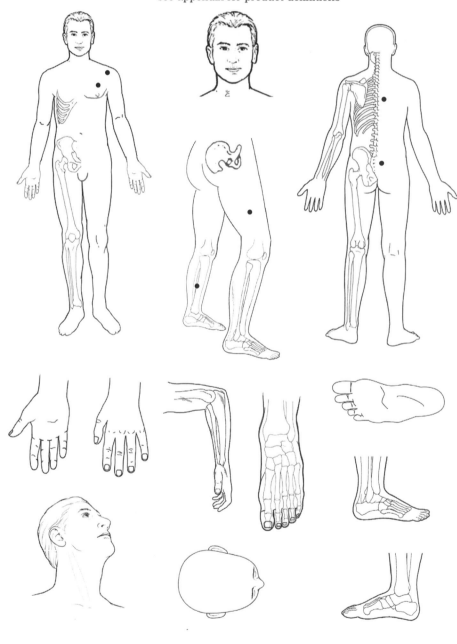

Jaundice

Emergency Nutritional Daily Menu	Maintenance Nutritional Daily Menu
Glyco: 6 tsp Phyto: 2 tsp Pre-Hormone: 6 tabs Cata-Blend: 4 tabs	Glyco: 2 tsp Phyto: 1 tsp Pre-Hormone: 3 tabs Cata-Blend: 4 tabs

see appendix for product definitions

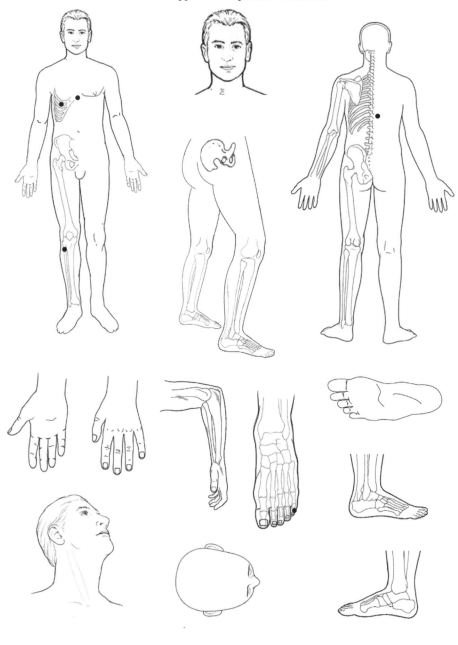

244

Jock Itch

Emergency Nutritional Daily Menu	Maintenance Nutritional Daily Menu
Glyco: 2 tsp Phyto: 1 tsp Pre-Hormone: 4 tabs Essentials: 4 tabs	Glyco: 1/2 tsp Phyto: 1/2 tsp Pre-Hormone: 3 tabs Essentials: 4 tabs

see appendix for product definitions

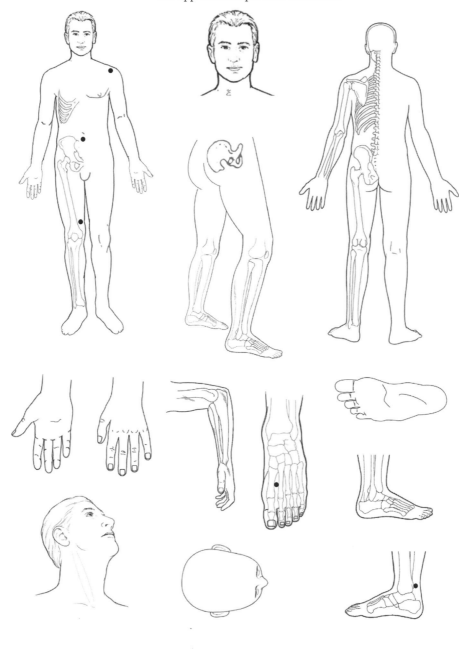

Joint pain (Multiple Sites)

Emergency Nutritional Daily Menu	Maintenance Nutritional Daily Menu
Glyco: 6 tsp Phyto: 1 tsp Pre-Hormone: 6 tabs Cata-Blend: 4 tabs	Glyco: 1 tsp Phyto: 1 tsp Pre-Hormone: 3 tabs Cata-Blend: 4 tabs

see appendix for product definitions

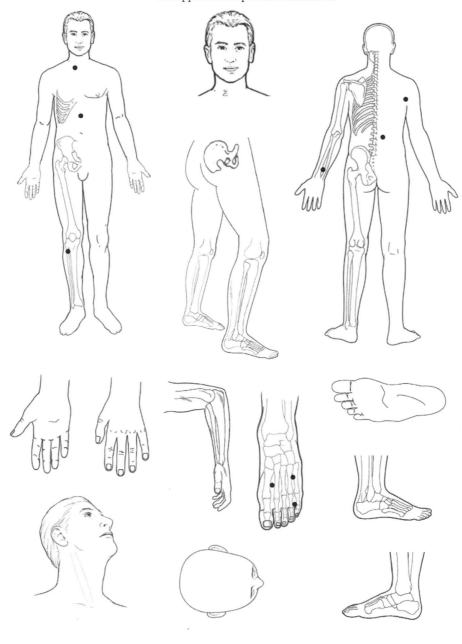

Juvenile Arthritis

Emergency Nutritional Daily Menu	Maintenance Nutritional Daily Menu
Glyco: 9 tsp Phyto: 2 tsp Pre-Hormone: 6 tabs Cata-Blend: 6 tabs	Glyco: 2 tsp Phyto: 1 tsp Pre-Hormone: 3 tabs Cata-Blend: 4 tabs

see appendix for product definitions

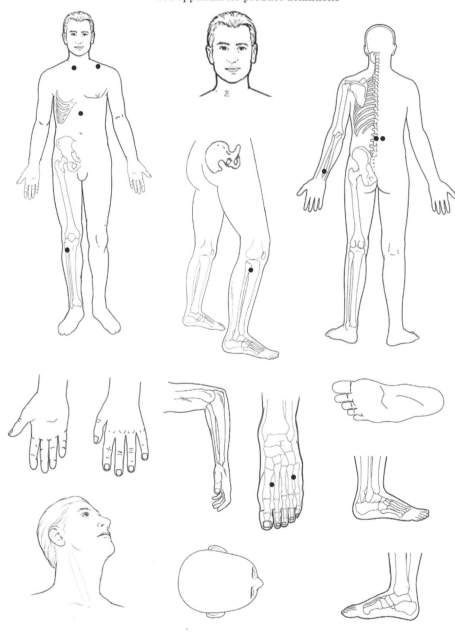

247

Kidney Detoxification

Emergency Nutritional Daily Menu	Maintenance Nutritional Daily Menu
Glyco: 9 tsp Phyto: 2 tsp Pre-Hormone: 6 tabs Cata-Blend: 4 tabs	Glyco: 1/2 tsp Phyto: 1/2 tsp Pre-Hormone: 3 tabs Cata-Blend: 4 tabs

see appendix for product definitions

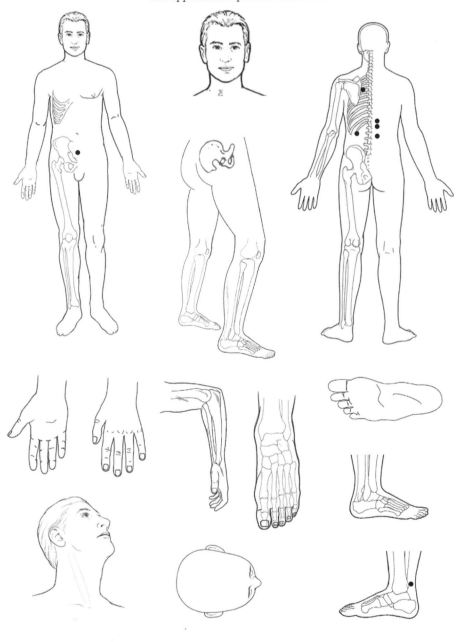

Kidney Infection

Emergency Nutritional Daily Menu	Maintenance Nutritional Daily Menu
Glyco: 3 tsp Phyto: 2 tsp Pre-Hormone: 4 tabs Cata-Blend: 4 tabs	Glyco: 1/2 tsp Phyto: 1/2 tsp Pre-Hormone: 3 tabs Cata-Blend: 4 tabs

see appendix for product definitions

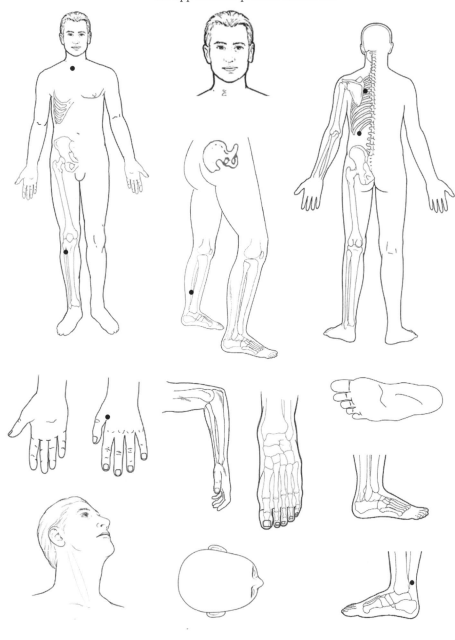

249

Labyrinthitis

Emergency Nutritional Daily Menu	Maintenance Nutritional Daily Menu
Glyco: 3 tsp Phyto: 1 tsp Pre-Hormone: 6 tabs Essentials: 4 tabs	Glyco: 1/2 tsp Phyto: 1/2 tsp Pre-Hormone: 3 tabs Essentials: 4 tabs

see appendix for product definitions

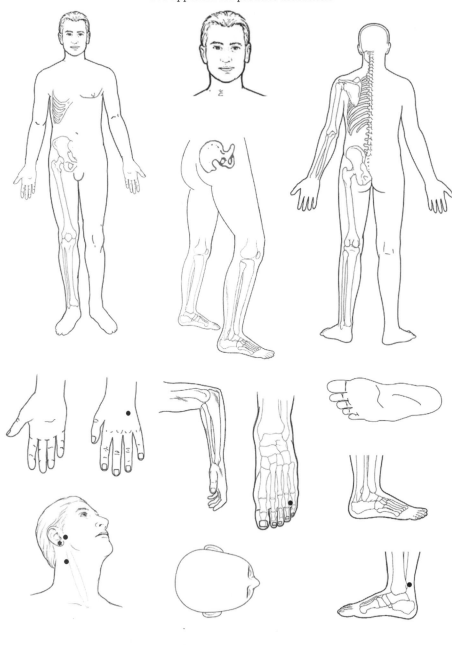

Laryngitis

Emergency Nutritional Daily Menu	Maintenance Nutritional Daily Menu
Glyco: 6 tsp Phyto: 2 tsp Pre-Hormone: 6 tabs Essentials: 4 tabs	Glyco: 1/2 tsp Phyto: 1/2 tsp Pre-Hormone: 3 tabs Essentials: 4 tabs

see appendix for product definitions

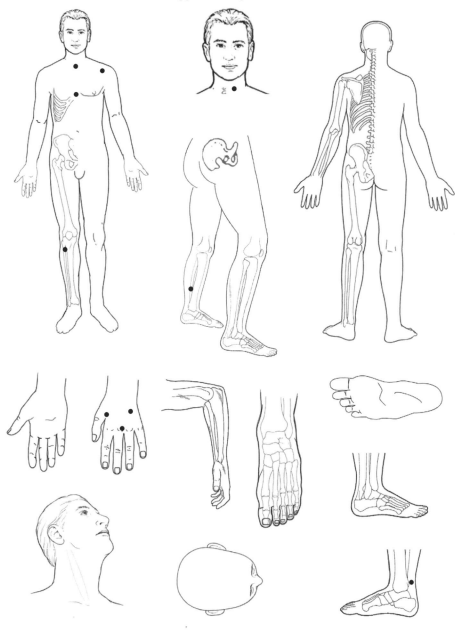

Leg Ulcers

Emergency Nutritional Daily Menu	Maintenance Nutritional Daily Menu
Glyco: 9 tsp Phyto: 2 tsp Pre-Hormone: 6 tabs Cata-Blend: 6 tabs	Glyco: 1 tsp Phyto: 1 tsp Pre-Hormone: 3 tabs Cata-Blend: 4 tabs

see appendix for product definitions

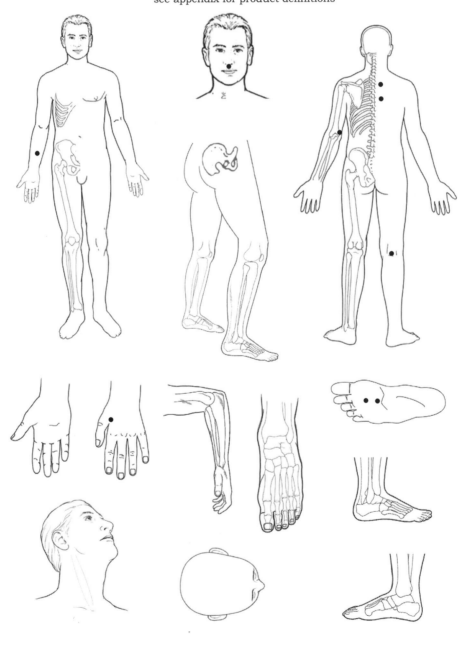

Leukemia

Emergency Nutritional Daily Menu	Maintenance Nutritional Daily Menu
Glyco: 12 tsp Phyto: 3 tsp Pre-Hormone: 4 tabs Cata-Blend: 6 tabs	Glyco: 3 tsp Phyto: 2 tsp Pre-Hormone: 3 tabs Cata-Blend: 4 tabs

see appendix for product definitions

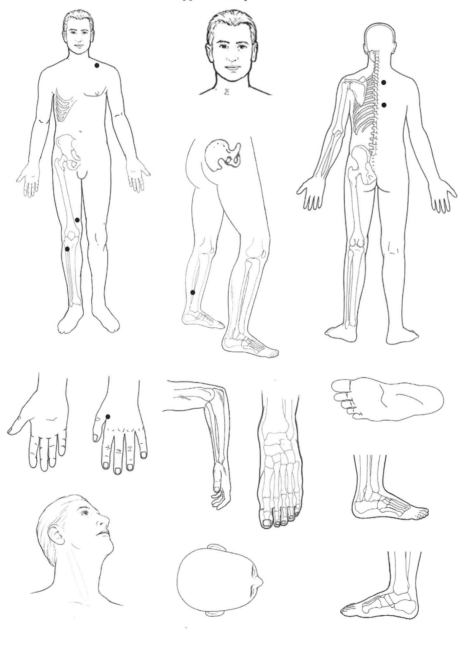

Liver Disease (Chronic)

Emergency Nutritional Daily Menu	Maintenance Nutritional Daily Menu
Glyco: 6 tsp Phyto: 2 tsp Pre-Hormone: 4 tabs Cata-Blend: 4 tabs	Glyco: 2 tsp Phyto: 1 tsp Pre-Hormone: 3 tabs Cata-Blend: 4 tabs

see appendix for product definitions

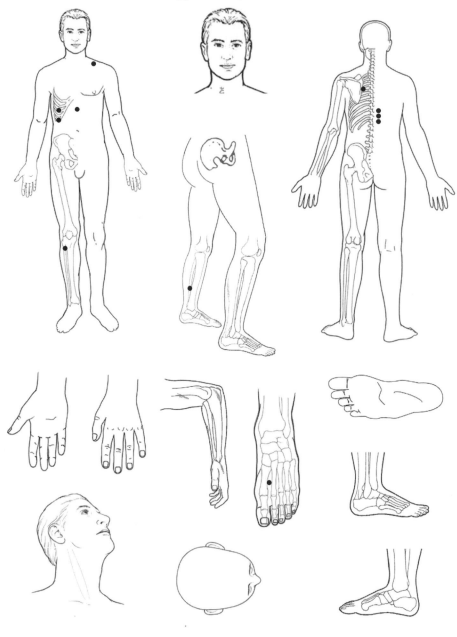

254

Lou Gehrig's Disease (ALS)

Emergency Nutritional Daily Menu	Maintenance Nutritional Daily Menu
Glyco: 12 tsp Phyto: 4 tsp Pre-Hormone: 6 tabs Cata-Blend: 6 tabs	Glyco: 3 tsp Phyto: 2 tsp Pre-Hormone: 4 tabs Cata-Blend: 6 tabs

see appendix for product definitions

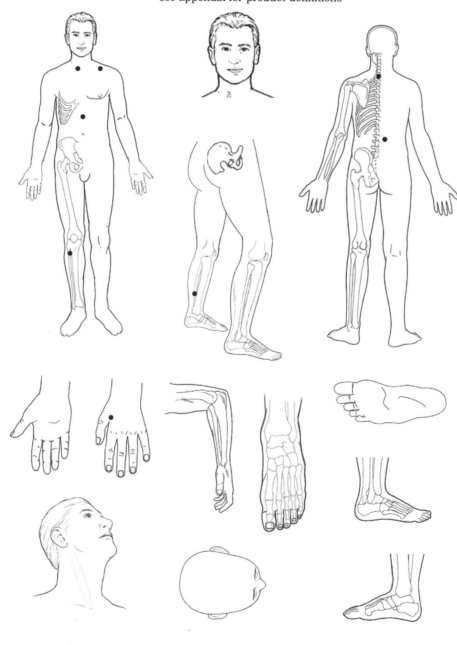

255

Low Blood Sugar

Emergency Nutritional Daily Menu	Maintenance Nutritional Daily Menu
Glyco: 6 tsp Phyto: 1 tsp Pre-Hormone: 6 tabs Cata-Blend: 4 tabs	Glyco: 1 tsp Phyto: 1 tsp Pre-Hormone: 4 tabs Cata-Blend: 4 tabs

see appendix for product definitions

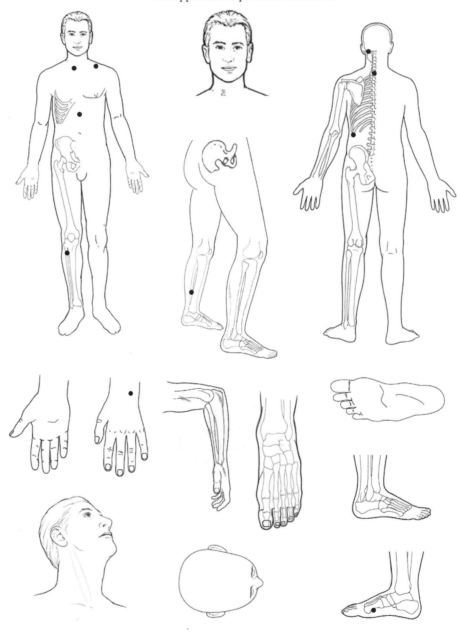

Lumbar Discitis

Emergency Nutritional Daily Menu	Maintenance Nutritional Daily Menu
Glyco: 9 tsp Phyto: 2 tsp Pre-Hormone: 6 tabs Cata-Blend: 4 tabs	Glyco: 1 tsp Phyto: 1/2 tsp Pre-Hormone: 4 tabs Cata-Blend: 4 tabs

see appendix for product definitions

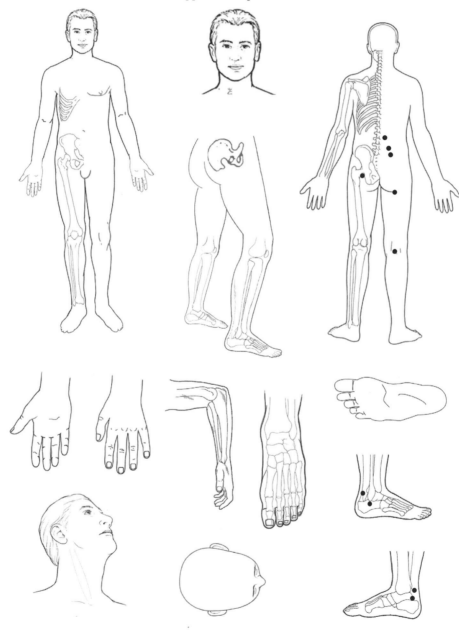

Lupus Erythematosis (SLE)

Emergency Nutritional Daily Menu	Maintenance Nutritional Daily Menu
Glyco: 9 tsp Phyto: 2 tsp Pre-Hormone: 4 tabs Cata-Blend: 6 tabs	Glyco: 2 tsp Phyto: 1 tsp Pre-Hormone: 3 tabs Cata-Blend: 6 tabs

see appendix for product definitions

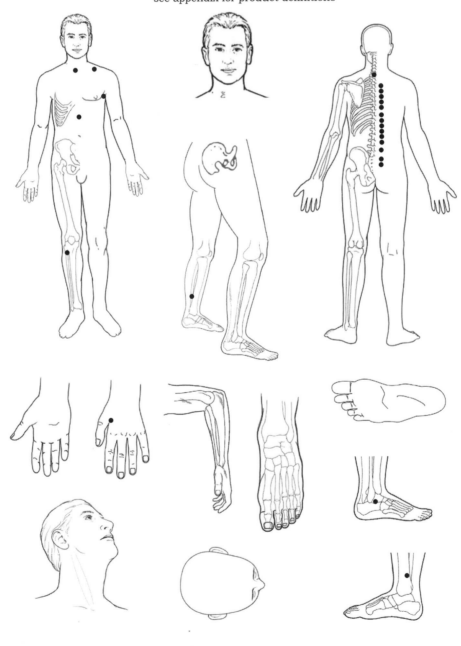

258

Lyme Disease

Emergency Nutritional Daily Menu	Maintenance Nutritional Daily Menu
Glyco: 9 tsp Phyto: 3 tsp Pre-Hormone: 6 tabs Cata-Blend: 6 tabs	Glyco: 2 tsp Phyto: 1 tsp Pre-Hormone: 3 tabs Cata-Blend: 6 tabs

see appendix for product definitions

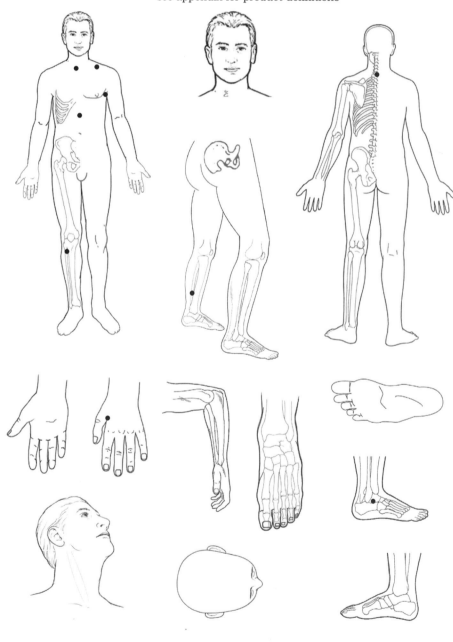

Lymph Nodes Swollen

Emergency Nutritional Daily Menu	Maintenance Nutritional Daily Menu
Glyco: 3 tsp Phyto: 2 tsp Pre-Hormone: 6 tabs Essentials: 4 tabs	Glyco: 1 tsp Phyto: 1/2 tsp Pre-Hormone: 3 tabs Essentials: 4 tabs

see appendix for product definitions

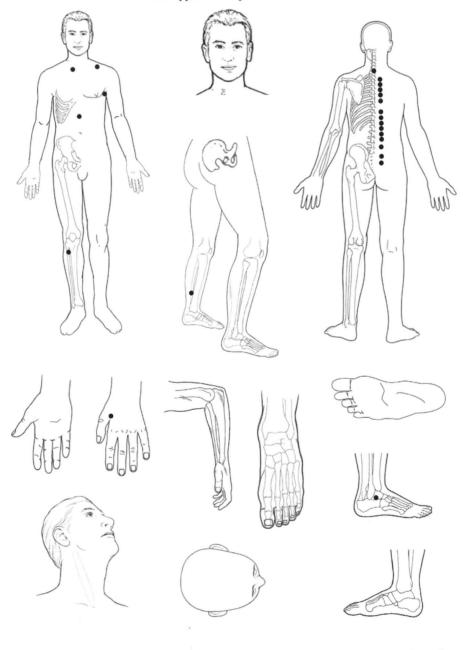

Lymphadenitis

Emergency Nutritional Daily Menu	Maintenance Nutritional Daily Menu
Glyco: 6 tsp Phyto: 2 tsp Pre-Hormone: 6 tabs Essentials: 4 tabs	Glyco: 1 tsp Phyto: 1/2 tsp Pre-Hormone: 3 tabs Essentials: 4 tabs

see appendix for product definitions

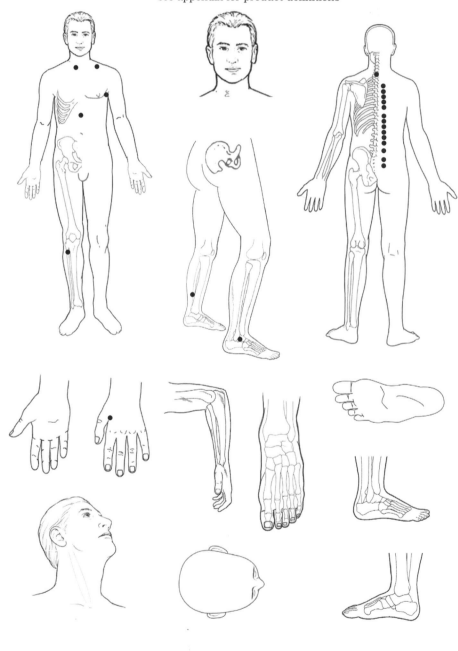

Lymphoma (Hodgkins)

Emergency Nutritional Daily Menu	Maintenance Nutritional Daily Menu
Glyco: 9 tsp Phyto: 4 tsp Pre-Hormone: 6 tabs Cata-Blend: 6 tabs	Glyco: 3 tsp Phyto: 2 tsp Pre-Hormone: 3 tabs Cata-Blend: 6 tabs

see appendix for product definitions

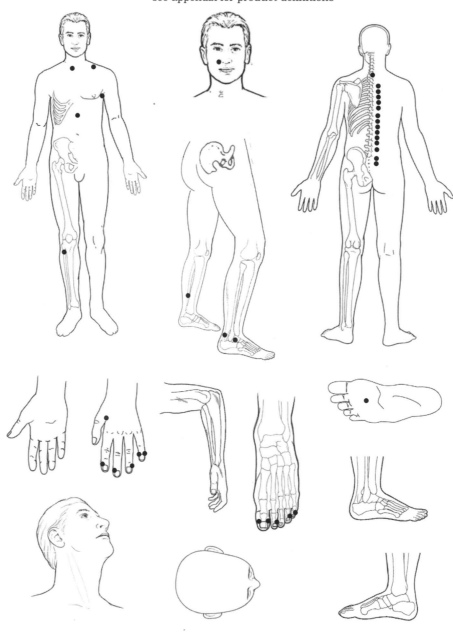

Macular Degeneration

Emergency Nutritional Daily Menu	Maintenance Nutritional Daily Menu
Glyco: 9 tsp Phyto: 3 tsp Pre-Hormone: 4 tabs Cata-Blend: 6 tabs	Glyco: 2 tsp Phyto: 2 tsp Pre-Hormone: 3 tabs Cata-Blend: 6 tabs

see appendix for product definitions

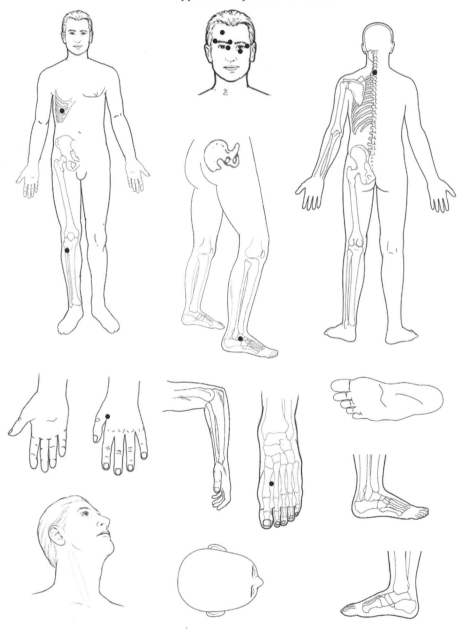

263

Malaria

Emergency Nutritional Daily Menu	Maintenance Nutritional Daily Menu
Glyco: 9 tsp Phyto: 2 tsp Pre-Hormone: 4 tabs Cata-Blend: 4 tabs	Glyco: 2 tsp Phyto: 1 tsp Pre-Hormone: 3 tabs Cata-Blend: 4 tabs

see appendix for product definitions

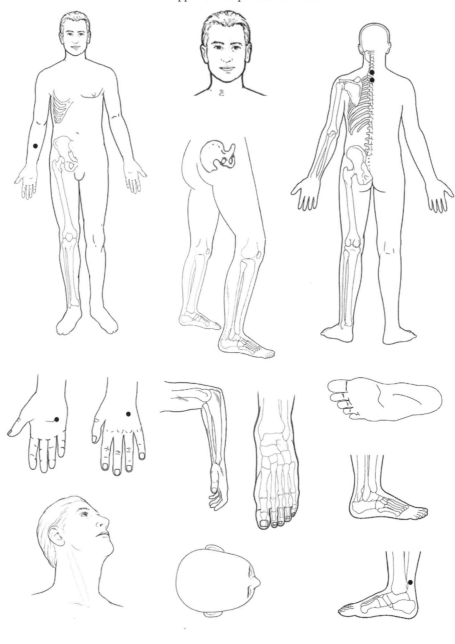

Malignant Melanoma

Emergency Nutritional Daily Menu	Maintenance Nutritional Daily Menu
Glyco: 12 tsp Phyto: 6 tsp Pre-Hormone: 6 tabs Cata-Blend: 6 tabs	Glyco: 3 tsp Phyto: 3 tsp Pre-Hormone: 3 tabs Cata-Blend: 6 tabs

see appendix for product definitions

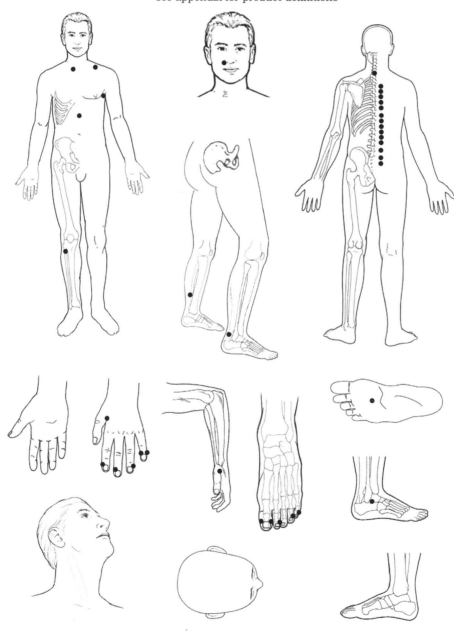

Mastitis

Emergency Nutritional Daily Menu	Maintenance Nutritional Daily Menu
Glyco: 6 tsp Phyto: 2 tsp Pre-Hormone: 4 tabs Cata-Blend: 4 tabs	Glyco: 2 tsp Phyto: 1/2 tsp Pre-Hormone: 3 tabs Cata-Blend: 4 tabs

see appendix for product definitions

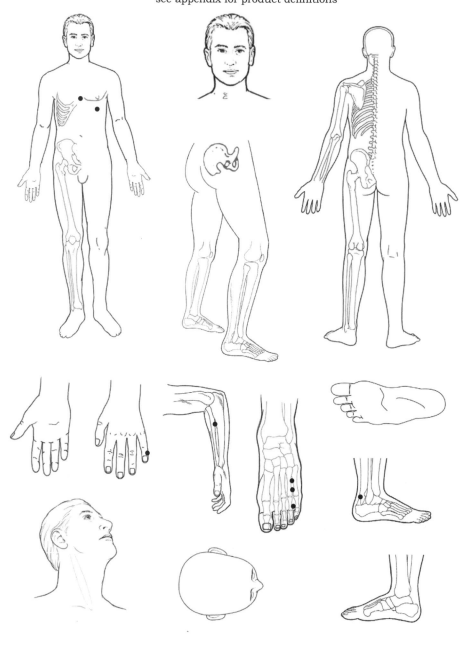

266

Measles

Emergency Nutritional Daily Menu	Maintenance Nutritional Daily Menu
Glyco: 3 tsp Phyto: 2 tsp Pre-Hormone: 4 tabs Essentials: 4 tabs	Glyco: 1/2 tsp Phyto: 1/2 tsp Pre-Hormone: 3 tabs Essentials: 4 tabs

see appendix for product definitions

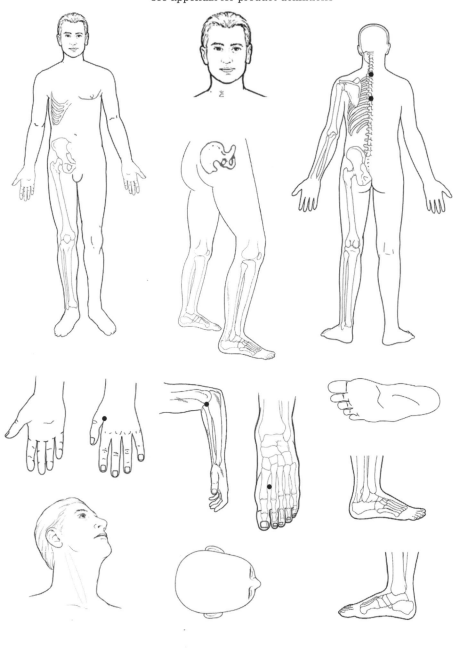

Meniere's Syndrome

Emergency Nutritional Daily Menu	Maintenance Nutritional Daily Menu
Glyco: 6 tsp Phyto: 2 tsp Pre-Hormone: 6 tabs Cata-Blend: 4 tabs	Glyco: 1 tsp Phyto: 1/2 tsp Pre-Hormone: 3 tabs Cata-Blend: 4 tabs

see appendix for product definitions

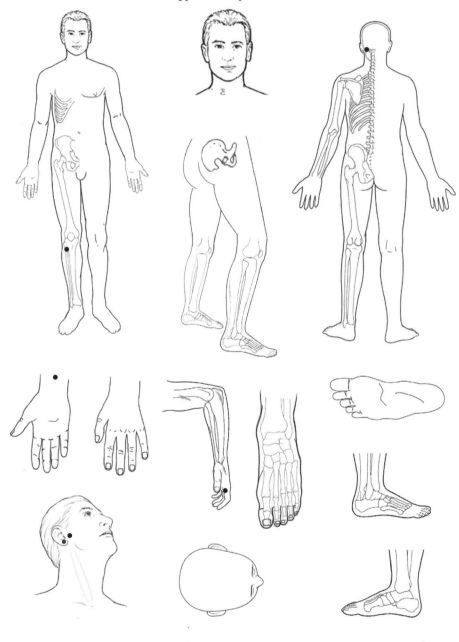

268

Meningitis

Emergency Nutritional Daily Menu	Maintenance Nutritional Daily Menu
Glyco: 12 tsp Phyto: 3 tsp Pre-Hormone: 6 tabs Cata-Blend: 6 tabs	Glyco: 1 tsp Phyto: 1/2 tsp Pre-Hormone: 3 tabs Cata-Blend: 4 tabs

see appendix for product definitions

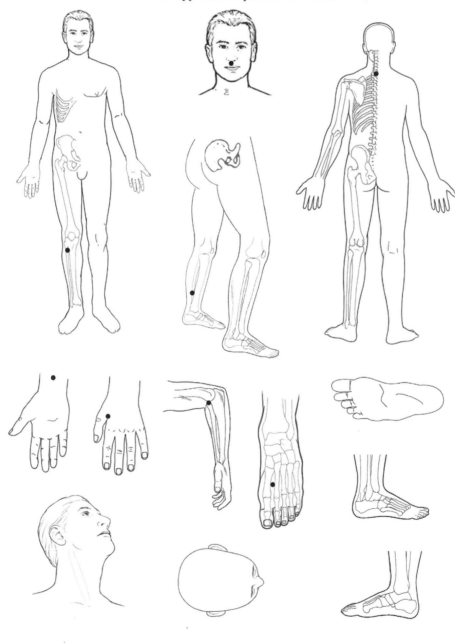

Menopausal Disorder

Emergency Nutritional Daily Menu	Maintenance Nutritional Daily Menu
Glyco: 3 tsp Phyto: 2 tsp Pre-Hormone: 4 tabs Essentials: 4 tabs	Glyco: 1 tsp Phyto: 1/2 tsp Pre-Hormone: 4 tabs Essentials: 4 tabs

see appendix for product definitions

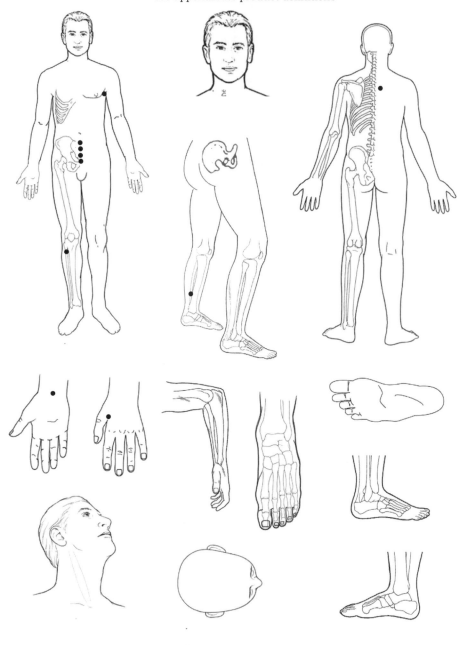

270

Menstrual Cramps (Dysmenorrhea)

Emergency Nutritional Daily Menu	Maintenance Nutritional Daily Menu
Glyco: 3 tsp Phyto: 1 tsp Pre-Hormone: 4 tabs Essentials: 4 tabs	Glyco: 1/2 tsp Phyto: 1/2 tsp Pre-Hormone: 4 tabs Essentials: 4 tabs

see appendix for product definitions

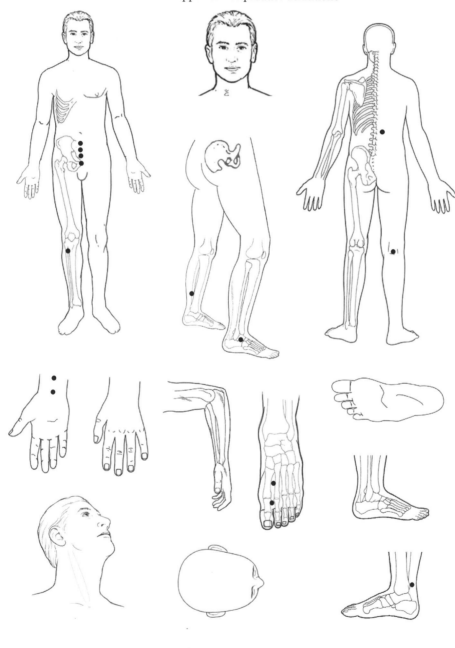

Mental Retardation

Emergency Nutritional Daily Menu	Maintenance Nutritional Daily Menu
Glyco: 9 tsp Phyto: 2 tsp Pre-Hormone: 6 tabs Cata-Blend: 4 tabs	Glyco: 2 tsp Phyto: 1 tsp Pre-Hormone: 4 tabs Cata-Blend: 4 tabs

see appendix for product definitions

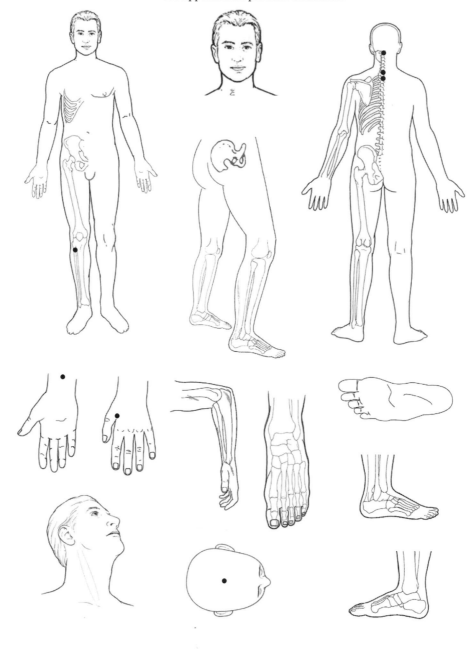

Mercury Detoxification

Emergency Nutritional Daily Menu	Maintenance Nutritional Daily Menu
Glyco: 12 tsp Phyto: 3 tsp Pre-Hormone: 6 tabs Cata-Blend: 6 tabs	Glyco: 2 tsp Phyto: 1 tsp Pre-Hormone: 3 tabs Cata-Blend: 4 tabs

see appendix for product definitions

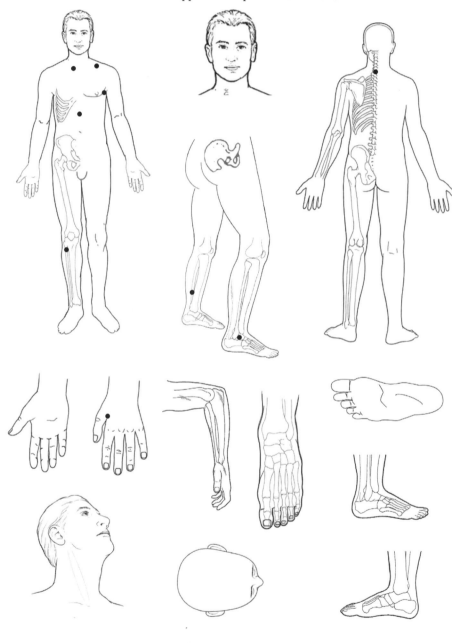

Metastatic Carcinoma

Emergency Nutritional Daily Menu	Maintenance Nutritional Daily Menu
Glyco: 12 tsp Phyto: 4 tsp Pre-Hormone: 6 tabs Cata-Blend: 6 tabs	Glyco: 3 tsp Phyto: 2 tsp Pre-Hormone: 4 tabs Cata-Blend: 6 tabs

see appendix for product definitions

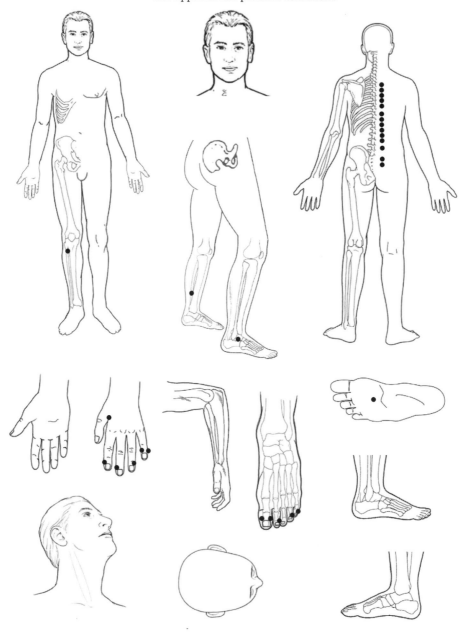

Migraine

Emergency Nutritional Daily Menu	Maintenance Nutritional Daily Menu
Glyco: 9 tsp Phyto: 2 tsp Pre-Hormone: 6 tabs Cata-Blend: 4 tabs	Glyco: 1 tsp Phyto: 1 tsp Pre-Hormone: 4 tabs Cata-Blend: 4 tabs

see appendix for product definitions

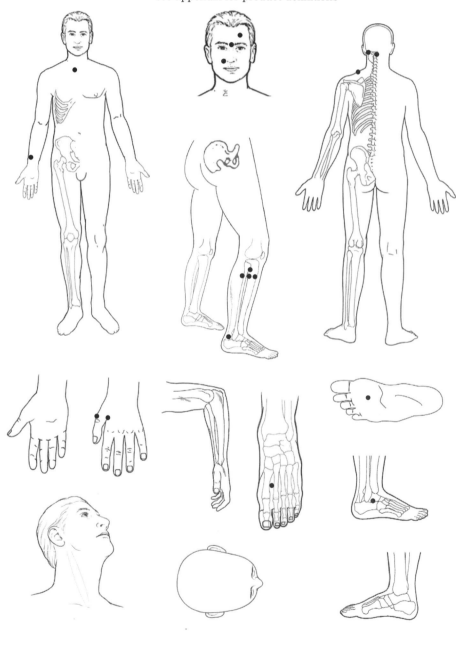

Mononucleosis

Emergency Nutritional Daily Menu	Maintenance Nutritional Daily Menu
Glyco: 9 tsp Phyto: 2 tsp Pre-Hormone: 4 tabs Cata-Blend: 4 tabs	Glyco: 1 tsp Phyto: 1 tsp Pre-Hormone: 3 tabs Cata-Blend: 4 tabs

see appendix for product definitions

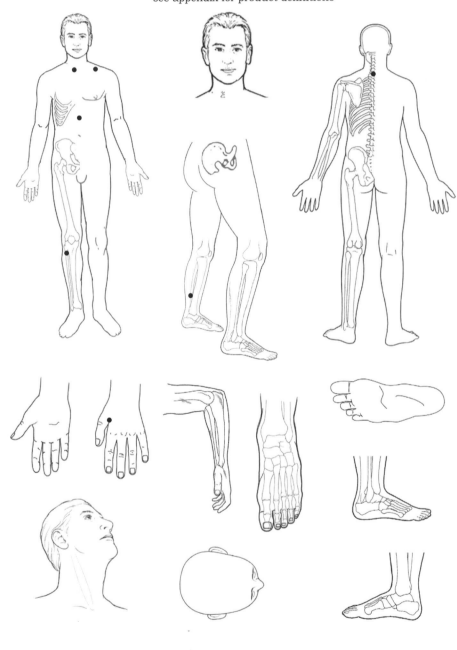

Mouth Sores

(apply soft laser to affect areas)

Emergency Nutritional Daily Menu	Maintenance Nutritional Daily Menu
Glyco: 6 tsp Phyto: 1 tsp Pre-Hormone: 4 tabs Essentials: 4 tabs	Glyco: 1/2 tsp Phyto: 1/2 tsp Pre-Hormone: 3 tabs Essentials: 4 tabs

see appendix for product definitions

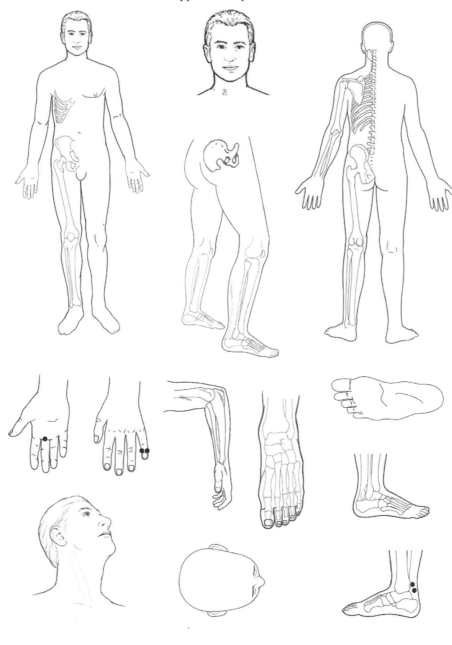

Multiple Myeloma

Emergency Nutritional Daily Menu	Maintenance Nutritional Daily Menu
Glyco: 12 tsp Phyto: 4 tsp Pre-Hormone: 6 tabs Cata-Blend: 6 tabs	Glyco: 3 tsp Phyto: 2 tsp Pre-Hormone: 4 tabs Cata-Blend: 6 tabs

see appendix for product definitions

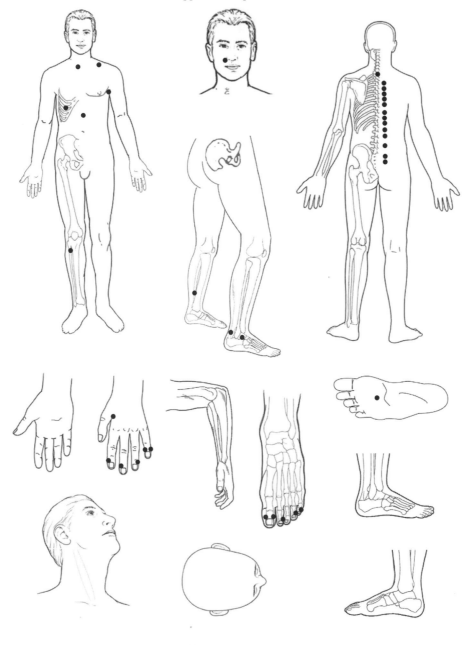

278

Multiple Sclerosis (MS)

Emergency Nutritional Daily Menu	Maintenance Nutritional Daily Menu
Glyco: 12 tsp Phyto: 4 tsp Pre-Hormone: 6 tabs Cata-Blend: 6 tabs	Glyco: 3 tsp Phyto: 2 tsp Pre-Hormone: 4 tabs Cata-Blend: 6 tabs

see appendix for product definitions

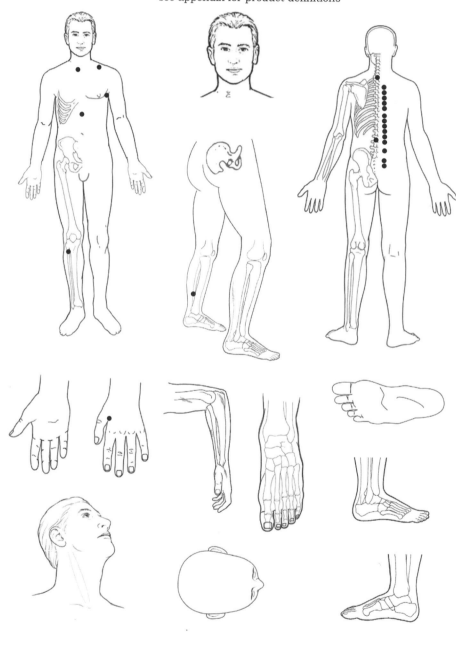

Mumps

Emergency Nutritional Daily Menu	Maintenance Nutritional Daily Menu
Glyco: 3 tsp Phyto: 2 tsp Pre-Hormone: 3 tabs Essentials: 4 tabs	Glyco: 1/2 tsp Phyto: 1/2 tsp Pre-Hormone: 3 tabs Essentials: 4 tabs

see appendix for product definitions

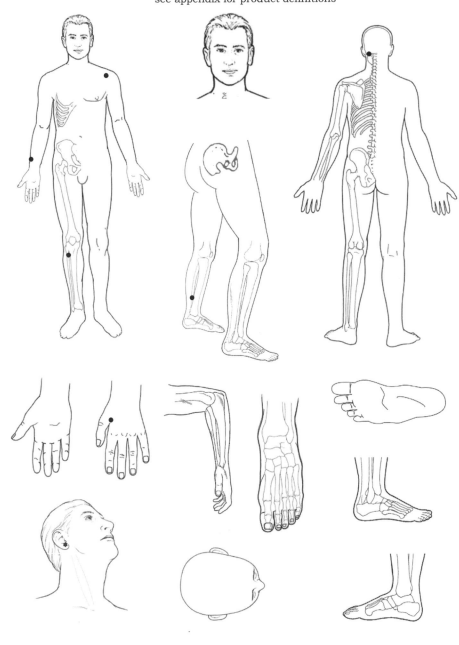

Myasthenia Gravis

Emergency Nutritional Daily Menu	Maintenance Nutritional Daily Menu
Glyco: 9 tsp Phyto: 1 tsp Pre-Hormone: 4 tabs Cata-Blend: 4 tabs	Glyco: 2 tsp Phyto: 1 tsp Pre-Hormone: 3 tabs Cata-Blend: 4 tabs

see appendix for product definitions

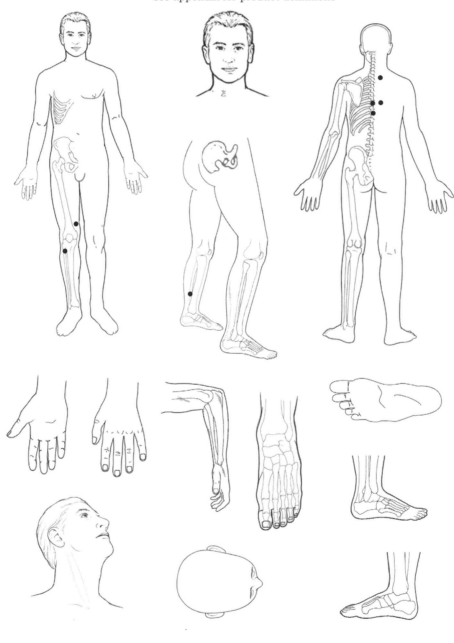

Myocardial Infarction (non-acute)

Emergency Nutritional Daily Menu	Maintenance Nutritional Daily Menu
Glyco: 9 tsp Phyto: 1 tsp Pre-Hormone: 6 tabs Cata-Blend: 6 tabs	Glyco: 2 tsp Phyto: 1 tsp Pre-Hormone: 3 tabs Cata-Blend: 4 tabs

see appendix for product definitions

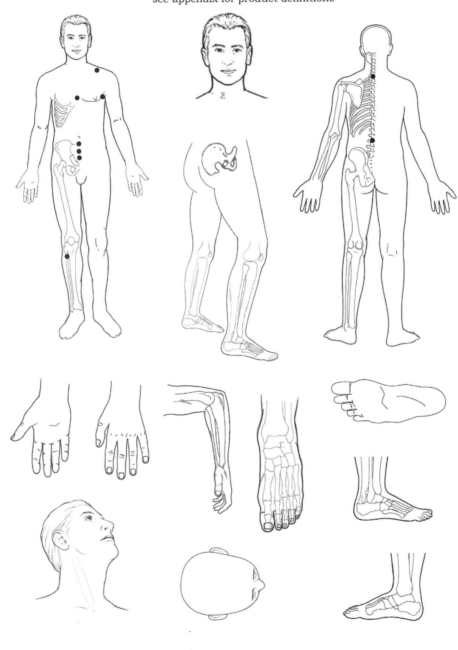

Myocarditis

Emergency Nutritional Daily Menu	Maintenance Nutritional Daily Menu
Glyco: 9 tsp Phyto: 1 tsp Pre-Hormone: 6 tabs Cata-Blend: 6 tabs	Glyco: 2 tsp Phyto: 1 tsp Pre-Hormone: 3 tabs Cata-Blend: 4 tabs

see appendix for product definitions

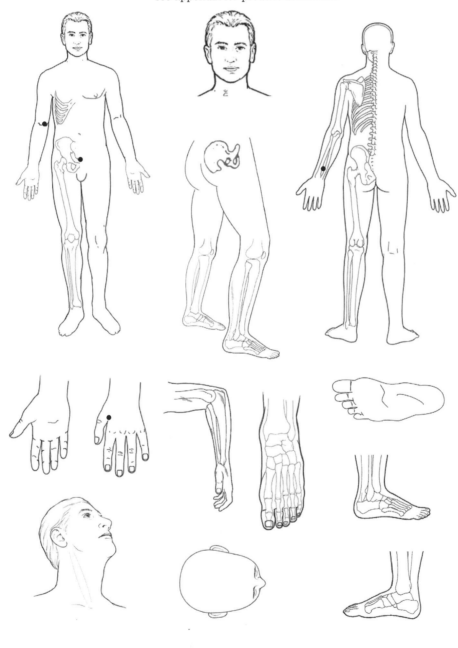

Myopathy

Emergency Nutritional Daily Menu	Maintenance Nutritional Daily Menu
Glyco: 9 tsp Phyto: 2 tsp Pre-Hormone: 6 tabs Cata-Blend: 6 tabs	Glyco: 2 tsp Phyto: 1 tsp Pre-Hormone: 3 tabs Cata-Blend: 4 tabs

see appendix for product definitions

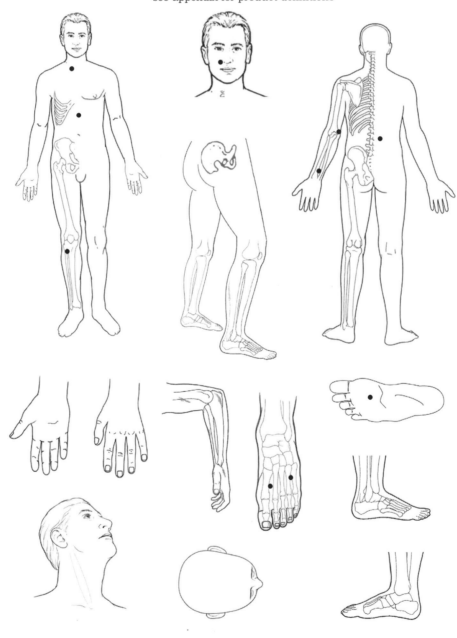

Narcolepsy

Emergency Nutritional Daily Menu	Maintenance Nutritional Daily Menu
Glyco: 6 tsp Phyto: 2 tsp Pre-Hormone: 6 tabs Cata-Blend: 4 tabs	Glyco: 2 tsp Phyto: 1 tsp Pre-Hormone: 3 tabs Cata-Blend: 4 tabs

see appendix for product definitions

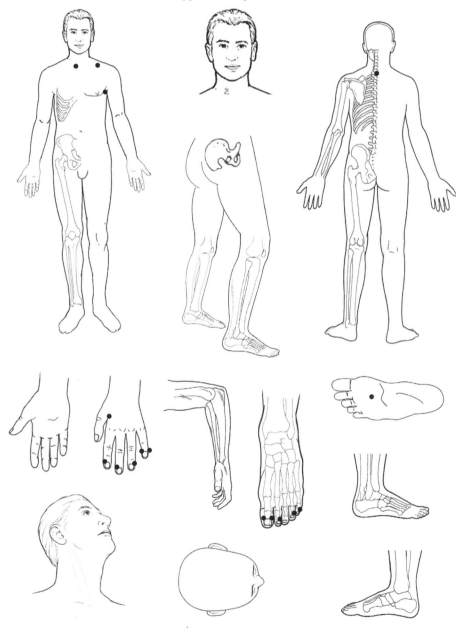

Nasal Polyp

Emergency Nutritional Daily Menu	Maintenance Nutritional Daily Menu
Glyco: 3 tsp Phyto: 1/2 tsp Pre-Hormone: 3 tabs Essentials: 4 tabs	Glyco: 1/2 tsp Phyto: 1/2 tsp Pre-Hormone: 3 tabs Essentials: 4 tabs

see appendix for product definitions

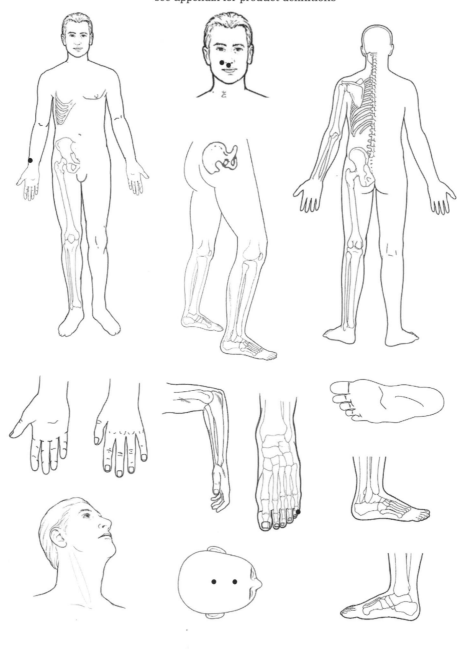

Nausea

Emergency Nutritional Daily Menu	Maintenance Nutritional Daily Menu
Glyco: 3 tsp Phyto: 1/2 tsp Pre-Hormone: 3 tabs Essentials: 4 tabs	Glyco: 1/2 tsp Phyto: 1/2 tsp Pre-Hormone: 3 tabs Essentials: 4 tabs

see appendix for product definitions

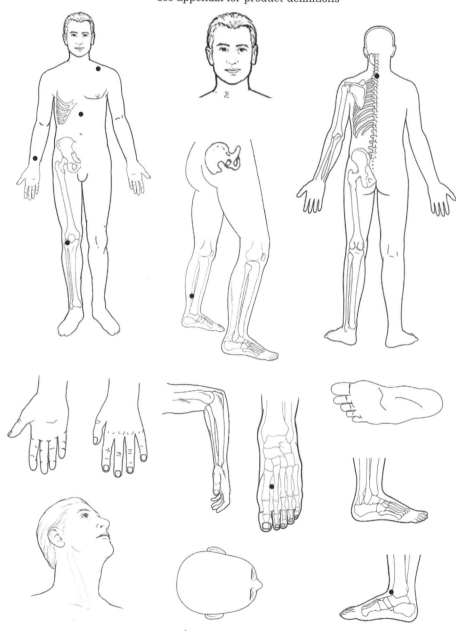

Nephritis

Emergency Nutritional Daily Menu	Maintenance Nutritional Daily Menu
Glyco: 9 tsp Phyto: 2 tsp Pre-Hormone: 3 tabs Essentials: 4 tabs	Glyco: 1/2 tsp Phyto: 1/2 tsp Pre-Hormone: 3 tabs Essentials: 4 tabs

see appendix for product definitions

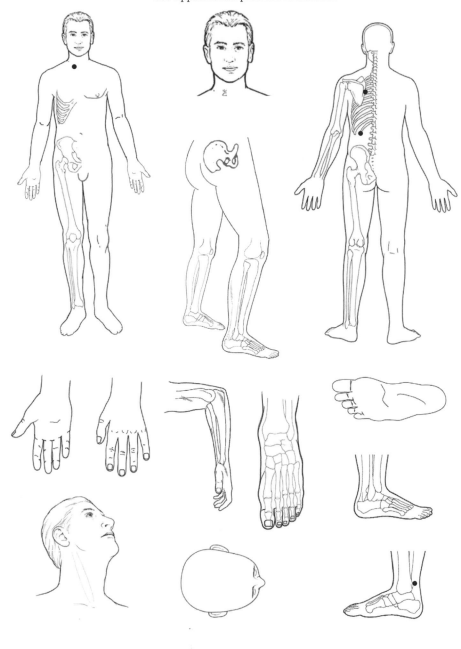

288

Neuralgia (Post-Herpetic)

Emergency Nutritional Daily Menu	Maintenance Nutritional Daily Menu
Glyco: 9 tsp Phyto: 1 tsp Pre-Hormone: 6 tabs Cata-Blend: 6 tabs	Glyco: 1 tsp Phyto: 1/2 tsp Pre-Hormone: 3 tabs Cata-Blend: 4 tabs

see appendix for product definitions

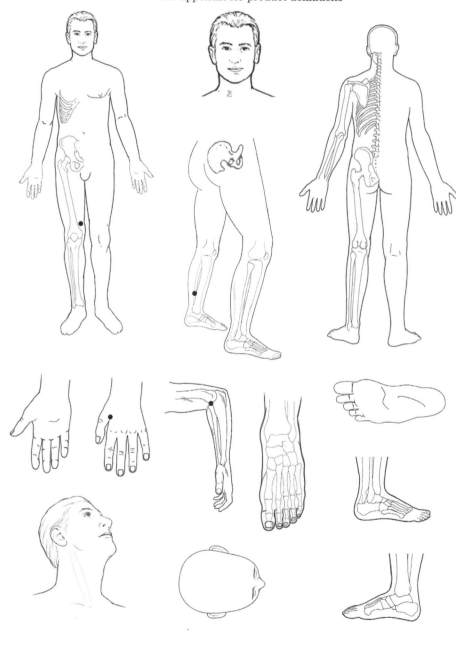

Neurogenic Bladder

Emergency Nutritional Daily Menu	Maintenance Nutritional Daily Menu
Glyco: 6 tsp Phyto: 1 tsp Pre-Hormone: 6 tabs Cata-Blend: 4 tabs	Glyco: 1 tsp Phyto: 1/2 tsp Pre-Hormone: 3 tabs Cata-Blend: 4 tabs

see appendix for product definitions

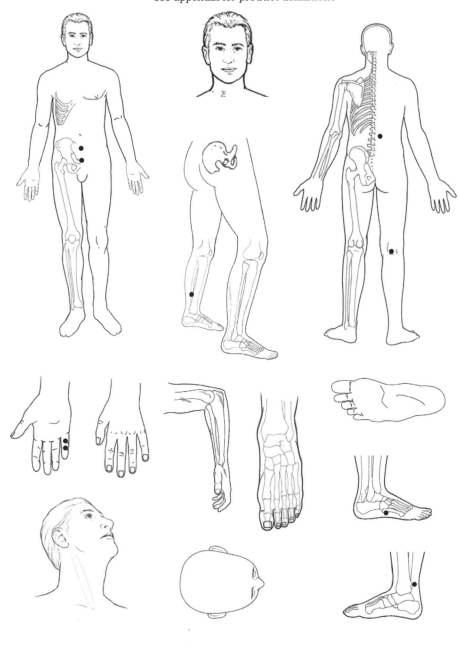

Neuromuscular Disorders

Emergency Nutritional Daily Menu	Maintenance Nutritional Daily Menu
Glyco: 12 tsp Phyto: 2 tsp Pre-Hormone: 6 tabs Cata-Blend: 6 tabs	Glyco: 2 tsp Phyto: 1 tsp Pre-Hormone: 4 tabs Cata-Blend: 4 tabs

see appendix for product definitions

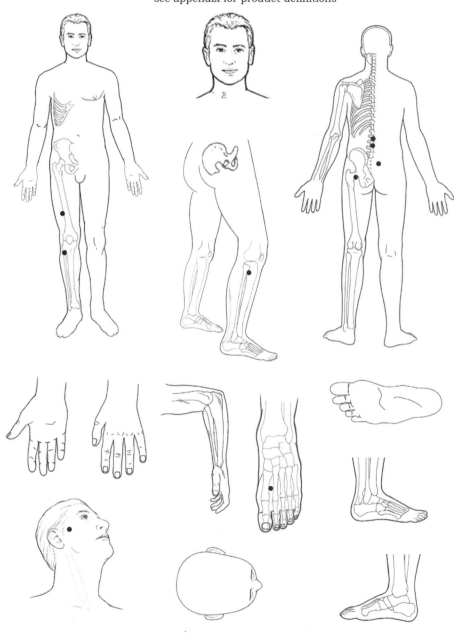

Night Sweats

Emergency Nutritional Daily Menu	Maintenance Nutritional Daily Menu
Glyco: 6 tsp Phyto: 1 tsp Pre-Hormone: 6 tabs Essentials: 4 tabs	Glyco: 1 tsp Phyto: 1/2 tsp Pre-Hormone: 3 tabs Essentials: 4 tabs

see appendix for product definitions

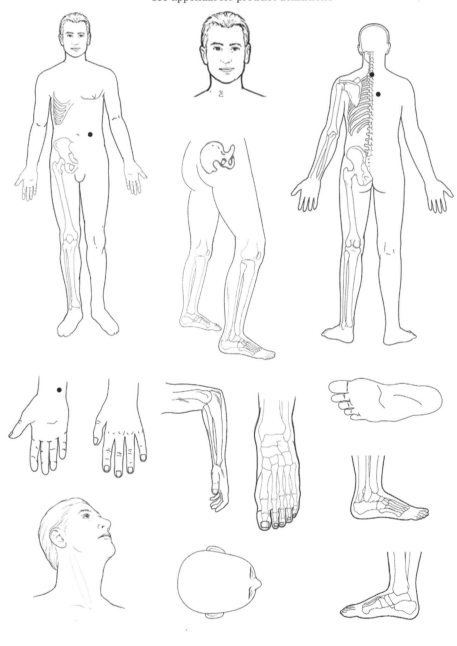

Obesity

Emergency Nutritional Daily Menu	Maintenance Nutritional Daily Menu
Glyco: 3 tsp Phyto: 1 tsp Pre-Hormone: 6 tabs Essentials: 6 tabs	Glyco: 1 tsp Phyto: 1 tsp Pre-Hormone: 4 tabs Essentials: 4 tabs

see appendix for product definitions

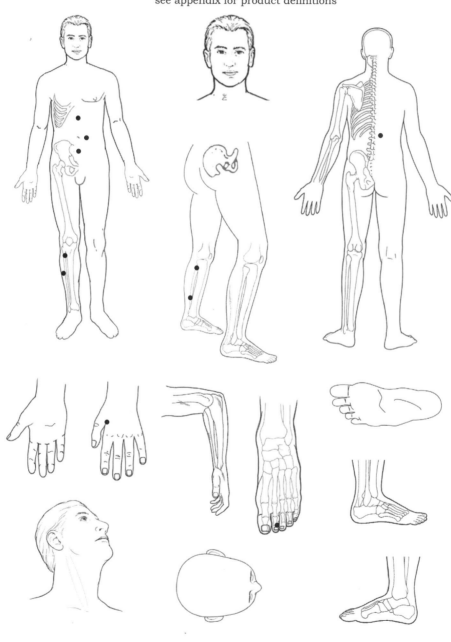

Optic Neuritis

Emergency Nutritional Daily Menu	Maintenance Nutritional Daily Menu
Glyco: 9 tsp Phyto: 2 tsp Pre-Hormone: 4 tabs Cata-Blend: 6 tabs	Glyco: 2 tsp Phyto: 1 tsp Pre-Hormone: 3 tabs Cata-Blend: 4 tabs

see appendix for product definitions

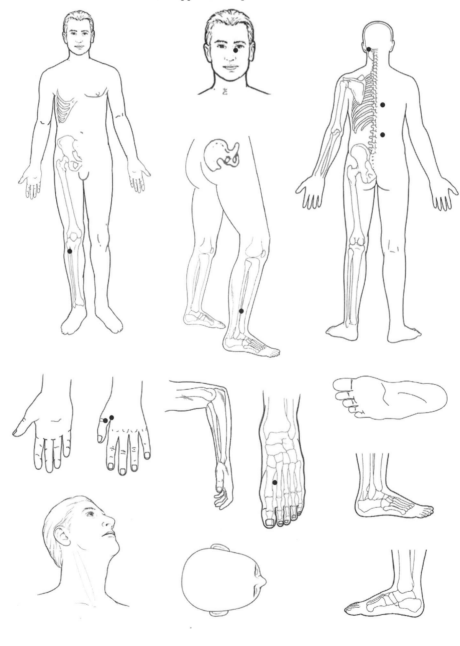

Osteoarthritis

Emergency Nutritional Daily Menu	Maintenance Nutritional Daily Menu
Glyco: 6 tsp Phyto: 1 tsp Pre-Hormone: 6 tabs Cata-Blend: 4 tabs	Glyco: 2 tsp Phyto: 1 tsp Pre-Hormone: 4 tabs Cata-Blend: 4 tabs

see appendix for product definitions

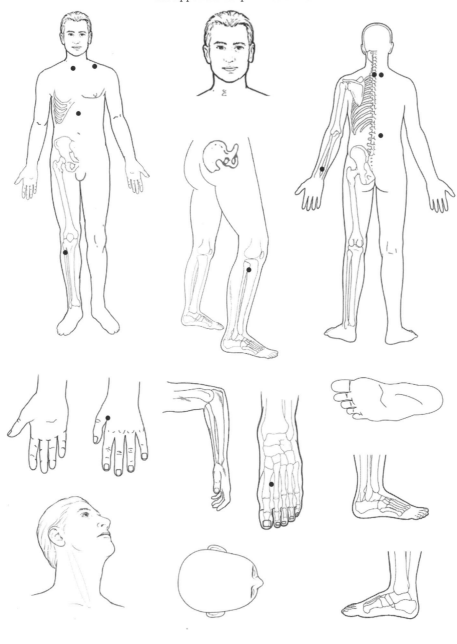

Osteomyelitis

Emergency Nutritional Daily Menu	Maintenance Nutritional Daily Menu
Glyco: 12 tsp Phyto: 2 tsp Pre-Hormone: 6 tabs Cata-Blend: 4 tabs	Glyco: 2 tsp Phyto: 1 tsp Pre-Hormone: 3 tabs Cata-Blend: 4 tabs

see appendix for product definitions

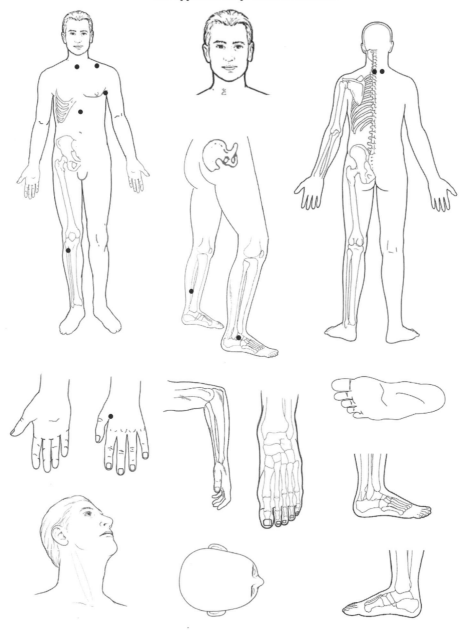

296

Osteoporosis

Emergency Nutritional Daily Menu	Maintenance Nutritional Daily Menu
Glyco: 3 tsp Phyto: 1 tsp Pre-Hormone: 6 tabs Cata-Blend: 4 tabs	Glyco: 1 tsp Phyto: 1 tsp Pre-Hormone: 4 tabs Cata-Blend: 4 tabs

see appendix for product definitions

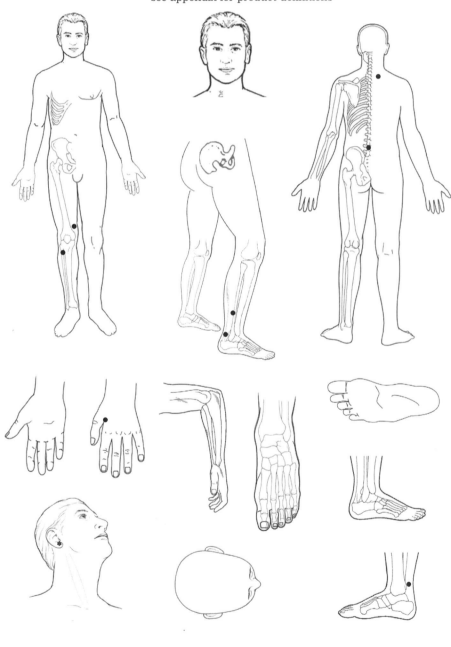

Otitis Media

Emergency Nutritional Daily Menu	Maintenance Nutritional Daily Menu
Glyco: 3 tsp Phyto: 1 tsp Pre-Hormone: 3 tabs Essentials: 4 tabs	Glyco: 1/2 tsp Phyto: 1/2 tsp Pre-Hormone: 3 tabs Essentials: 4 tabs

see appendix for product definitions

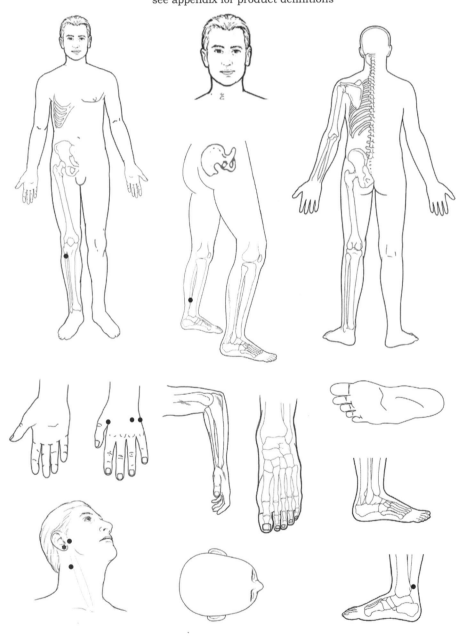

Ovaries (Infection)

Emergency Nutritional Daily Menu	Maintenance Nutritional Daily Menu
Glyco: 3 tsp Phyto: 1 tsp Pre-Hormone: 4 tabs Essentials: 4 tabs	Glyco: 1/2 tsp Phyto: 1/2 tsp Pre-Hormone: 3 tabs Essentials: 4 tabs

see appendix for product definitions

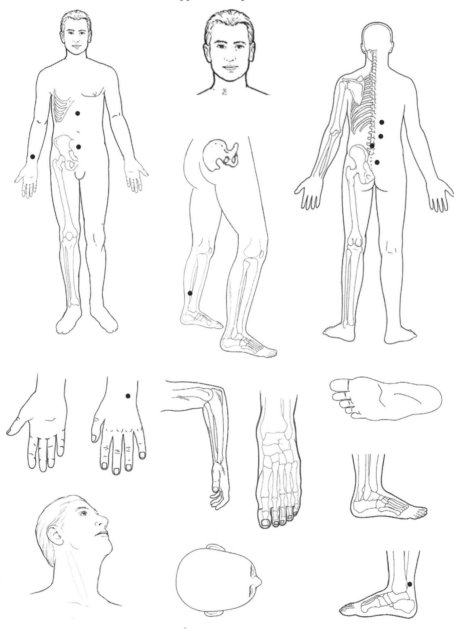

Pain (Generalized)

Emergency Nutritional Daily Menu	Maintenance Nutritional Daily Menu
Glyco: 6 tsp Phyto: 1 tsp Pre-Hormone: 6 tabs Cata-Blend: 4 tabs	Glyco: 1 tsp Phyto: 1/2 tsp Pre-Hormone: 4 tabs Cata-Blend: 4 tabs

see appendix for product definitions

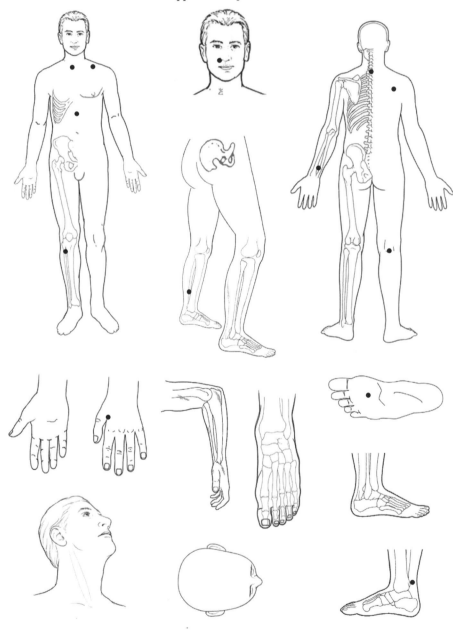

300

Pain (pleuritic)

Emergency Nutritional Daily Menu	Maintenance Nutritional Daily Menu
Glyco: 6 tsp Phyto: 1 tsp Pre-Hormone: 4 tabs Essentials: 4 tabs	Glyco: 1 tsp Phyto: 1/2 tsp Pre-Hormone: 4 tabs Essentials: 4 tabs

see appendix for product definitions

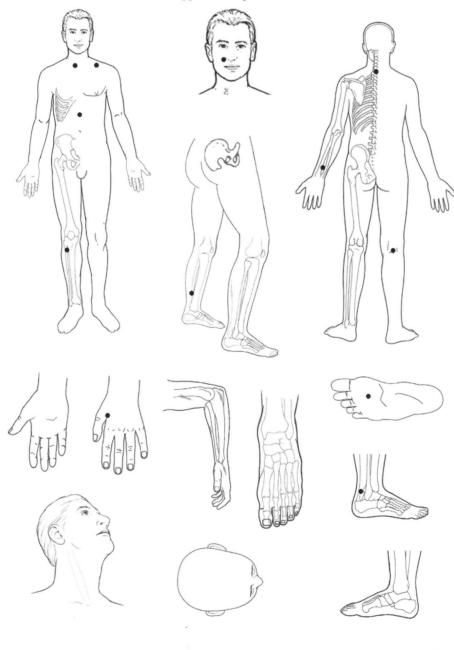

Palpitations

Emergency Nutritional Daily Menu	Maintenance Nutritional Daily Menu
Glyco: 6 tsp Phyto: 1 tsp Pre-Hormone: 3 tabs Cata-Blend: 4 tabs	Glyco: 1 tsp Phyto: 1/2 tsp Pre-Hormone: 3 tabs Cata-Blend: 4 tabs

see appendix for product definitions

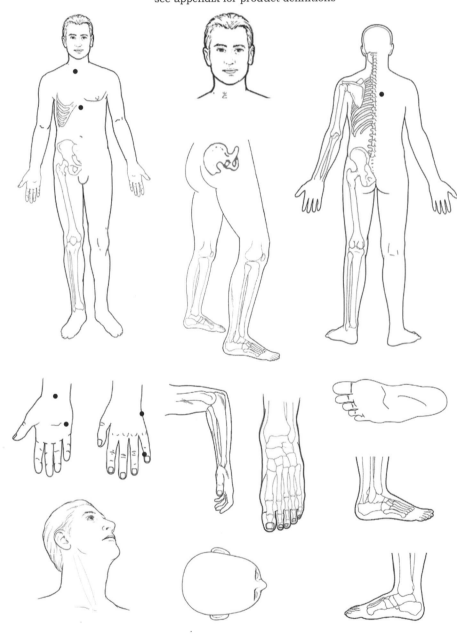

Pancreatitis (chronic)

Emergency Nutritional Daily Menu	Maintenance Nutritional Daily Menu
Glyco: 6 tsp Phyto: 1 tsp Pre-Hormone: 3 tabs Cata-Blend: 4 tabs	Glyco: 2 tsp Phyto: 1 tsp Pre-Hormone: 3 tabs Cata-Blend: 4 tabs

see appendix for product definitions

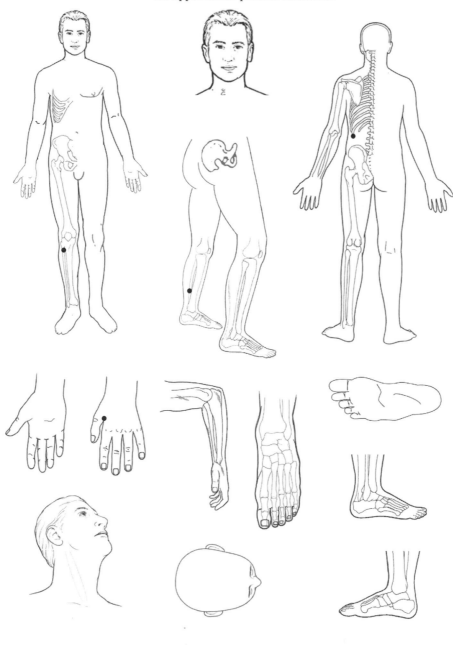

Panic Disorder

Emergency Nutritional Daily Menu	Maintenance Nutritional Daily Menu
Glyco: 6 tsp Phyto: 1/2 tsp Pre-Hormone: 6 tabs Cata-Blend: 4 tabs	Glyco: 2 tsp Phyto: 1/2 tsp Pre-Hormone: 3 tabs Cata-Blend: 4 tabs

see appendix for product definitions

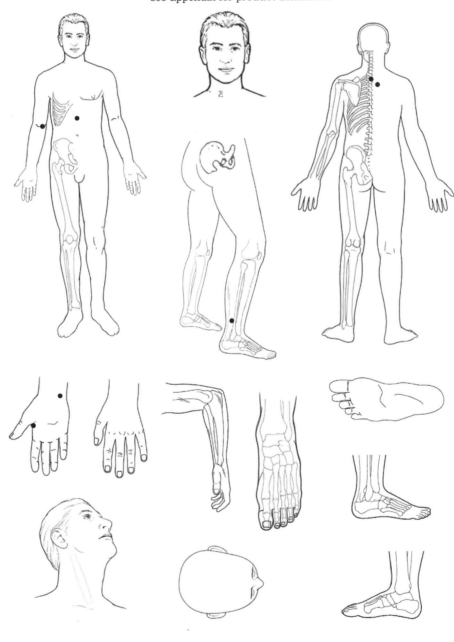

Paraplegia

(stimulate listed spinal points 2 vertebrae above and below injury)

Emergency Nutritional Daily Menu	Maintenance Nutritional Daily Menu
Glyco: 9 tsp Phyto: 2 tsp Pre-Hormone: 6 tabs Cata-Blend: 6 tabs	Glyco: 2 tsp Phyto: 1 tsp Pre-Hormone: 3 tabs Cata-Blend: 4 tabs

see appendix for product definitions

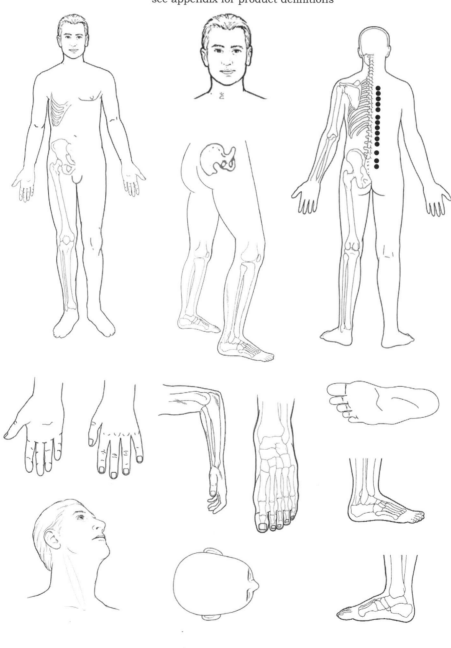

Parkinson's Disease

Emergency Nutritional Daily Menu	Maintenance Nutritional Daily Menu
Glyco: 3 tsp Phyto: 2 tsp Pre-Hormone: 6 tabs Cata-Blend: 4 tabs	Glyco: 3 tsp Phyto: 2 tsp Pre-Hormone: 3 tabs Cata-Blend: 4 tabs

see appendix for product definitions

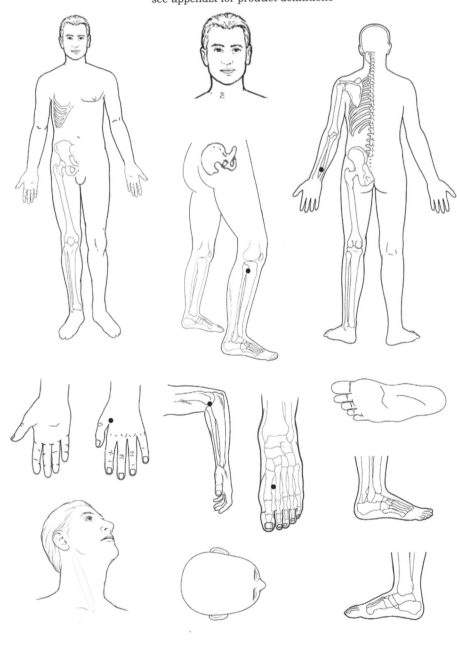

Pelvic Inflammatory Disease (PID)

Emergency Nutritional Daily Menu	Maintenance Nutritional Daily Menu
Glyco: 3 tsp Phyto: 1 tsp Pre-Hormone: 4 tabs Cata-Blend: 4 tabs	Glyco: 1 tsp Phyto: 1 tsp Pre-Hormone: 3 tabs Cata-Blend: 4 tabs

see appendix for product definitions

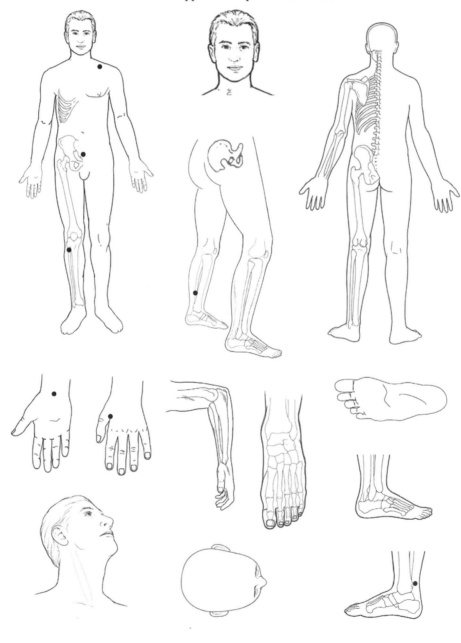

Peptic Ulcers

Emergency Nutritional Daily Menu	Maintenance Nutritional Daily Menu
Glyco: 6 tsp Phyto: 1 tsp Pre-Hormone: 4 tabs Cata-Blend: 4 tabs	Glyco: 1 tsp Phyto: 1 tsp Pre-Hormone: 3 tabs Cata-Blend: 4 tabs

see appendix for product definitions

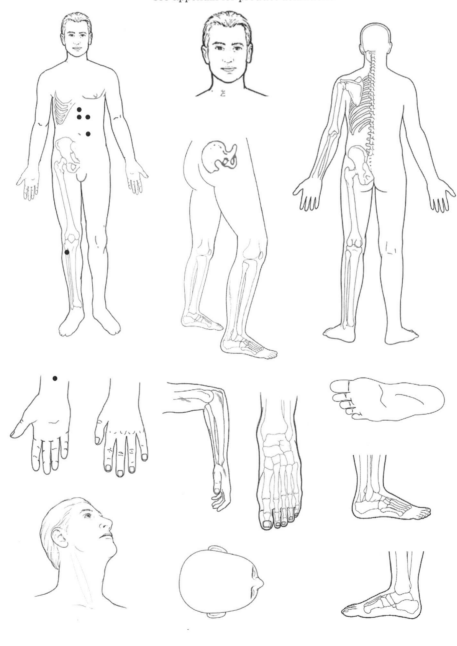

Peripheral Vascular Disease

Emergency Nutritional Daily Menu	Maintenance Nutritional Daily Menu
Glyco: 9 tsp Phyto: 2 tsp Pre-Hormone: 6 tabs Cata-Blend: 6 tabs	Glyco: 2 tsp Phyto: 1 tsp Pre-Hormone: 3 tabs Cata-Blend: 4 tabs

see appendix for product definitions

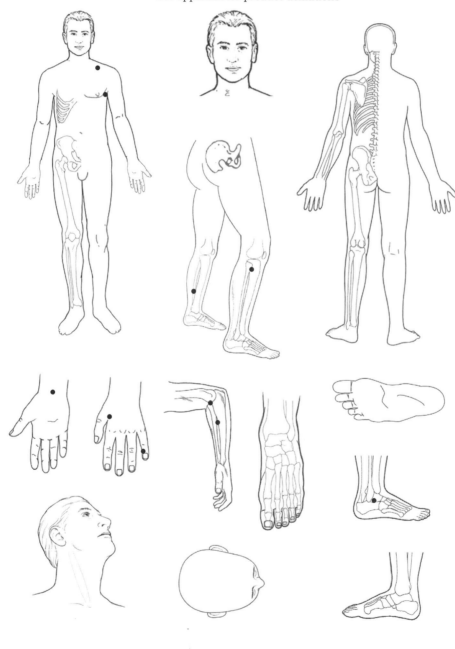

Pharyngitis (Sore Throat)

Emergency Nutritional Daily Menu	Maintenance Nutritional Daily Menu
Glyco: 3 tsp Phyto: 1 tsp Pre-Hormone: 3 tabs Essentials: 4 tabs	Glyco: 1/2 tsp Phyto: 1/2 tsp Pre-Hormone: 3 tabs Essentials: 4 tabs

see appendix for product definitions

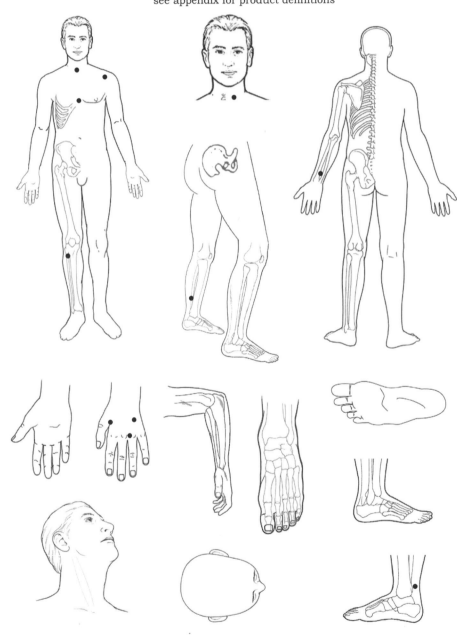

Pinkeye

Emergency Nutritional Daily Menu	Maintenance Nutritional Daily Menu
Glyco: 3 tsp Phyto: 1 tsp Pre-Hormone: 3 tabs Essentials: 4 tabs	Glyco: 1/2 tsp Phyto: 1/2 tsp Pre-Hormone: 3 tabs Essentials: 4 tabs

see appendix for product definitions

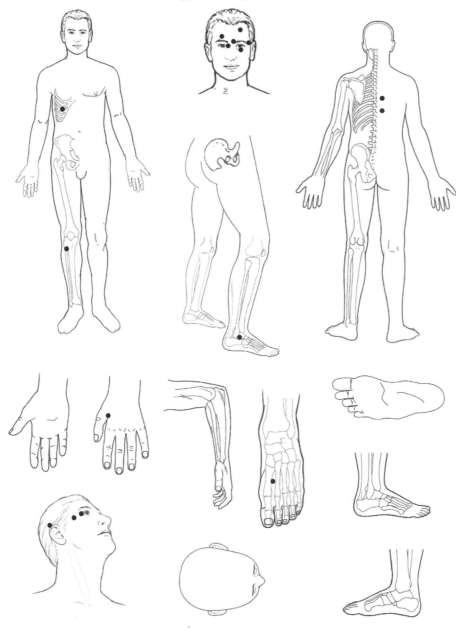

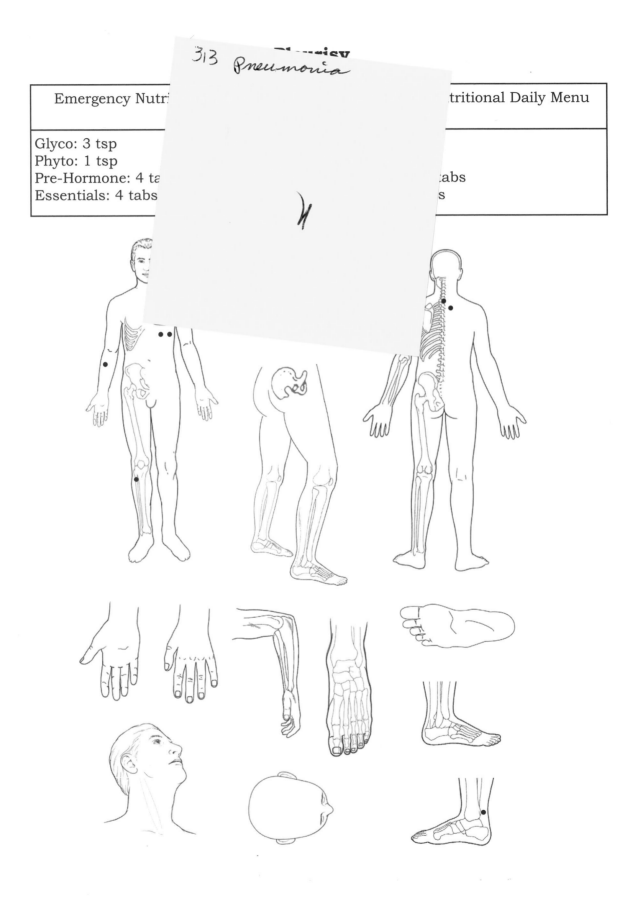

313 Pneumonia

Emergency Nutri[...]   [...]tritional Daily Menu

Glyco: 3 tsp
Phyto: 1 tsp
Pre-Hormone: 4 ta[...]   [...]tabs
Essentials: 4 tabs

Pneumonia

Emergency Nutritional Daily Menu	Maintenance Nutritional Daily Menu
Glyco: 6 tsp Phyto: 2 tsp Pre-Hormone: 4 tabs Essentials: 6 tabs	Glyco: 1/2 tsp Phyto: 1/2 tsp Pre-Hormone: 3 tabs Essentials: 4 tabs

see appendix for product definitions

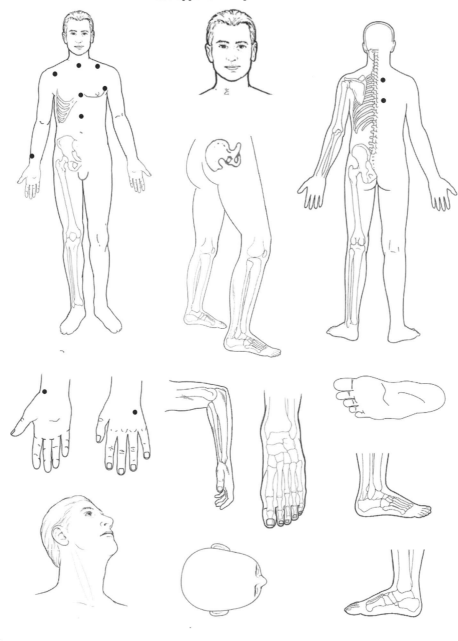

Polio

Emergency Nutritional Daily Menu	Maintenance Nutritional Daily Menu
Glyco: 9 tsp Phyto: 2 tsp Pre-Hormone: 6 tabs Cata-Blend: 4 tabs	Glyco: 3 tsp Phyto: 2 tsp Pre-Hormone: 3 tabs Cata-Blend: 4 tabs

see appendix for product definitions

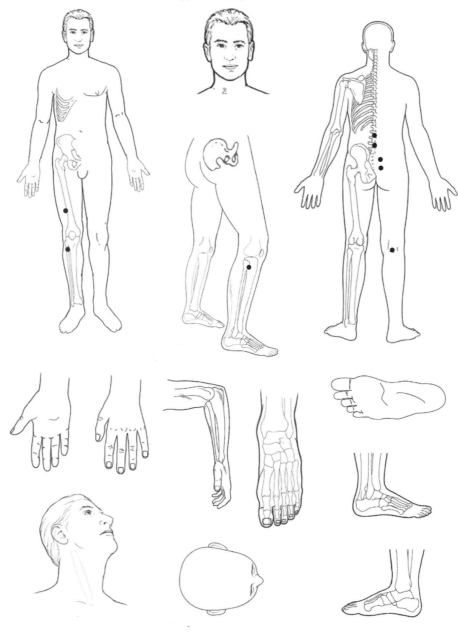

314

Polymyalgia Rheumatica

Emergency Nutritional Daily Menu	Maintenance Nutritional Daily Menu
Glyco: 12 tsp Phyto: 2 tsp Pre-Hormone: 6 tabs Cata-Blend: 6 tabs	Glyco: 3 tsp Phyto: 2 tsp Pre-Hormone: 4 tabs Cata-Blend: 4 tabs

see appendix for product definitions

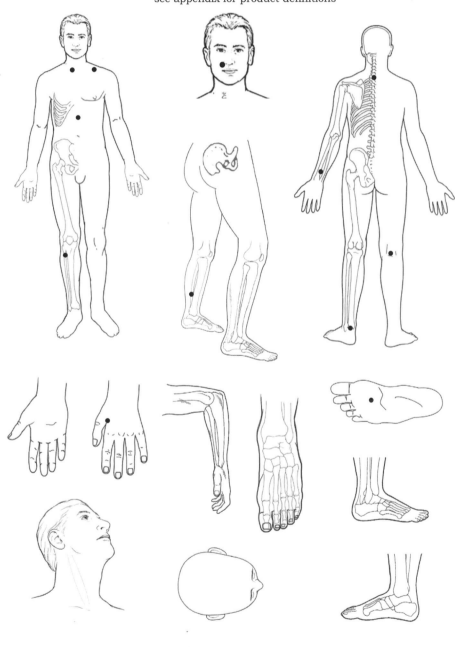

Premenstrual Syndrome (PMS)

Emergency Nutritional Daily Menu	Maintenance Nutritional Daily Menu
Glyco: 3 tsp Phyto: 1 tsp Pre-Hormone: 6 tabs Cata-Blend: 4 tabs	Glyco: 1 tsp Phyto: 1 tsp Pre-Hormone: 4 tabs Cata-Blend: 4 tabs

see appendix for product definitions

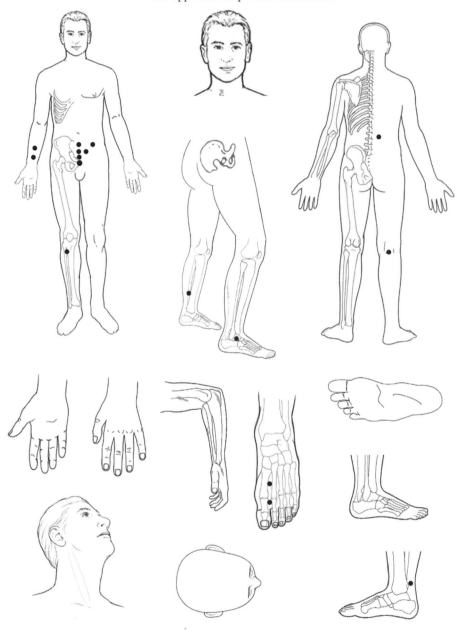

Prostatitis

Emergency Nutritional Daily Menu	Maintenance Nutritional Daily Menu
Glyco: 3 tsp Phyto: 2 tsp Pre-Hormone: 4 tabs Cata-Blend: 4 tabs	Glyco: 1 tsp Phyto: 1 tsp Pre-Hormone: 4 tabs Cata-Blend: 4 tabs

see appendix for product definitions

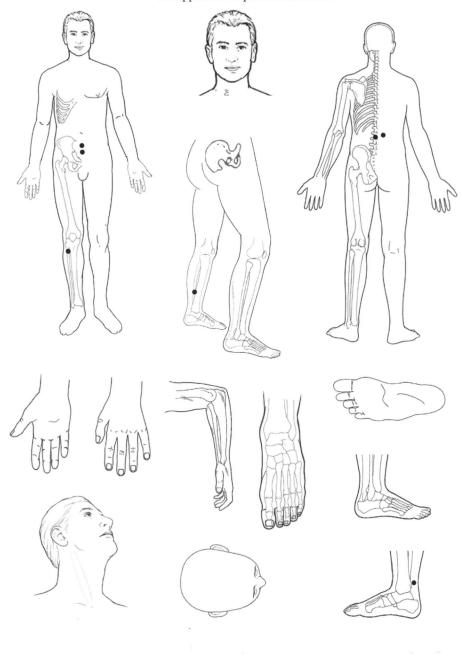

Pruritis

Emergency Nutritional Daily Menu	Maintenance Nutritional Daily Menu
Glyco: 3 tsp Phyto: 1 tsp Pre-Hormone: 6 tabs Cata-Blend: 4 tabs	Glyco: 1 tsp Phyto: 1/2 tsp Pre-Hormone: 4 tabs Cata-Blend: 4 tabs

see appendix for product definitions

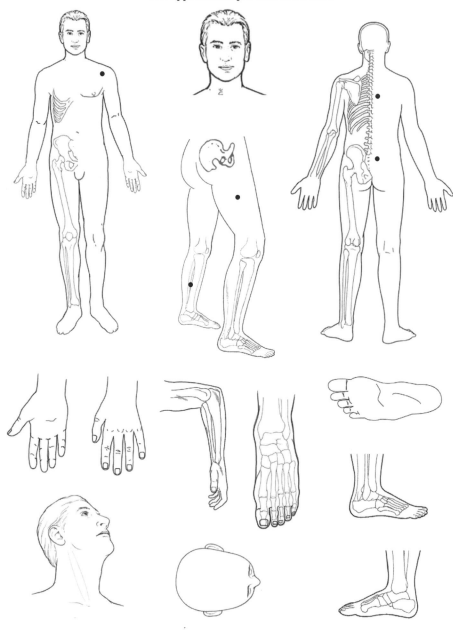

318

Psoriasis

(soft laser on affected areas)

Emergency Nutritional Daily Menu	Maintenance Nutritional Daily Menu
Glyco: 9 tsp Phyto: 1 tsp Pre-Hormone: 6 tabs Cata-Blend: 4 tabs	Glyco: 1 tsp Phyto: 1 tsp Pre-Hormone: 4 tabs Cata-Blend: 4 tabs

see appendix for product definitions

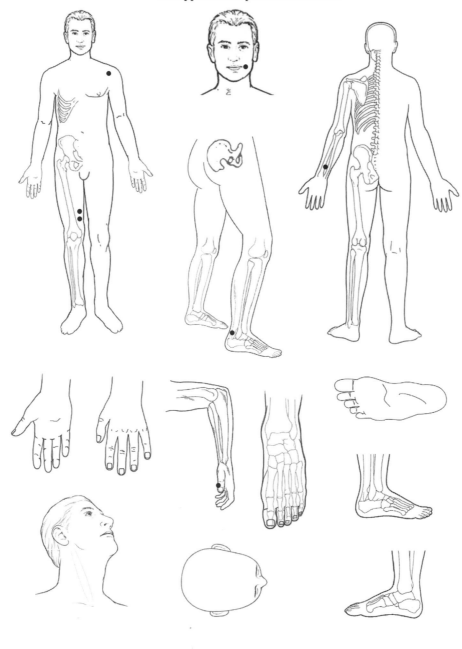

Psoriatic Arthritis

Emergency Nutritional Daily Menu	Maintenance Nutritional Daily Menu
Glyco: 9 tsp Phyto: 1 tsp Pre-Hormone: 6 tabs Cata-Blend: 6 tabs	Glyco: 2 tsp Phyto: 1 tsp Pre-Hormone: 4 tabs Cata-Blend: 4 tabs

see appendix for product definitions

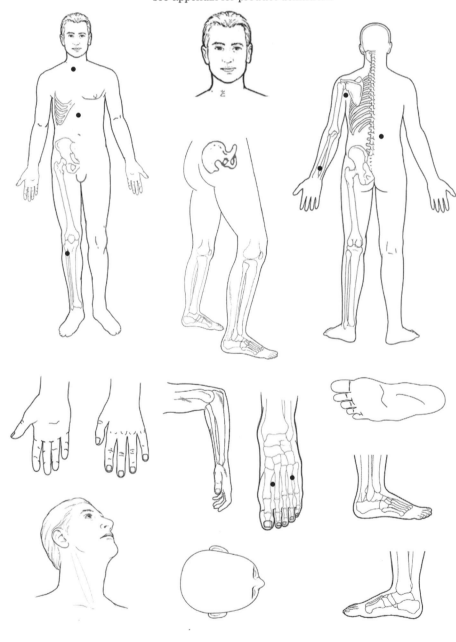

320

Pulmonary Fibrosis

Emergency Nutritional Daily Menu	Maintenance Nutritional Daily Menu
Glyco: 9 tsp Phyto: 2 tsp Pre-Hormone: 6 tabs Cata-Blend: 4 tabs	Glyco: 3 tsp Phyto: 2 tsp Pre-Hormone: 3 tabs Cata-Blend: 4 tabs

see appendix for product definitions

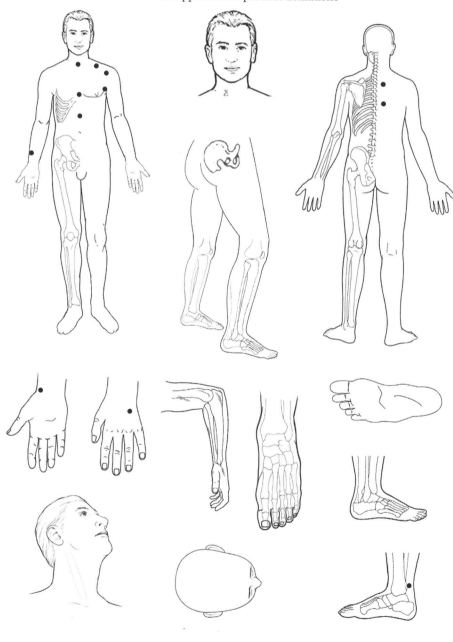

321

Pulmonary Hypertension

Emergency Nutritional Daily Menu	Maintenance Nutritional Daily Menu
Glyco: 6 tsp Phyto: 3 tsp Pre-Hormone: 4 tabs Cata-Blend: 4 tabs	Glyco: 2 tsp Phyto: 2 tsp Pre-Hormone: 3 tabs Cata-Blend: 4 tabs

see appendix for product definitions

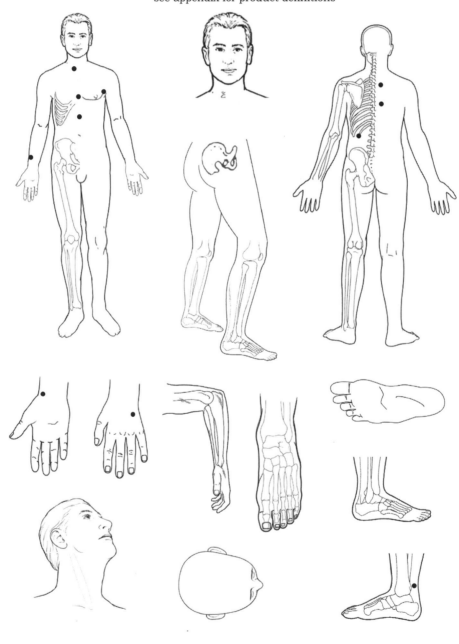

Pyelonephritis

Emergency Nutritional Daily Menu	Maintenance Nutritional Daily Menu
Glyco: 6 tsp Phyto: 1 tsp Pre-Hormone: 4 tabs Essentials: 4 tabs	Glyco: 1 tsp Phyto: 1 tsp Pre-Hormone: 3 tabs Essentials: 4 tabs

see appendix for product definitions

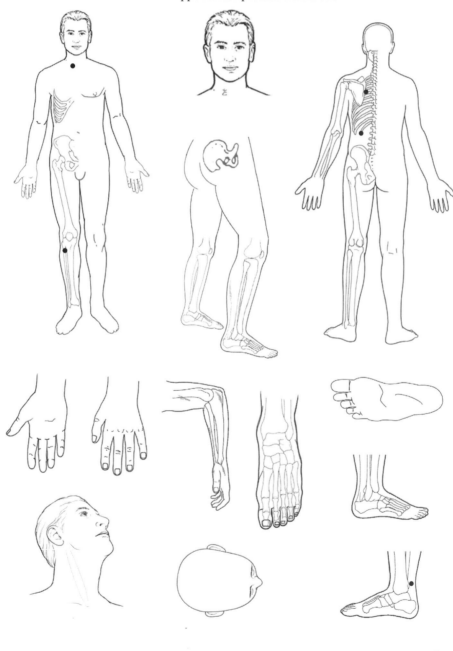

323

Rash

Emergency Nutritional Daily Menu	Maintenance Nutritional Daily Menu
Glyco: 3 tsp Phyto: 1/2 tsp Pre-Hormone: 4 tabs Essentials: 4 tabs	Glyco: 1/2 tsp Phyto: 1/2 tsp Pre-Hormone: 3 tabs Essentials: 4 tabs

see appendix for product definitions

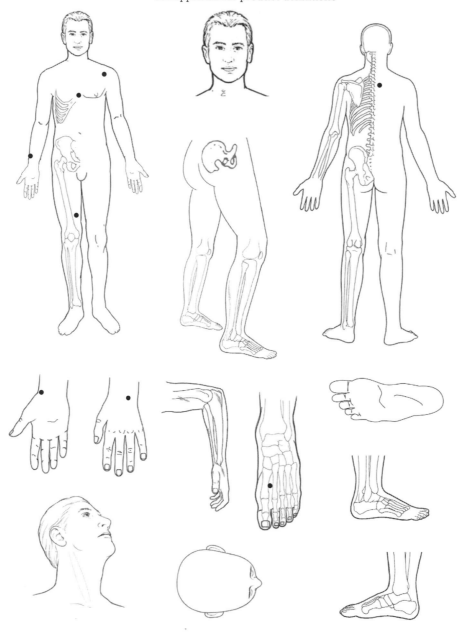

Raynaud's Syndrome

Emergency Nutritional Daily Menu	Maintenance Nutritional Daily Menu
Glyco: 6 tsp Phyto: 1 tsp Pre-Hormone: 6 tabs Cata-Blend: 4 tabs	Glyco: 2 tsp Phyto: 1 tsp Pre-Hormone: 3 tabs Cata-Blend: 4 tabs

see appendix for product definitions

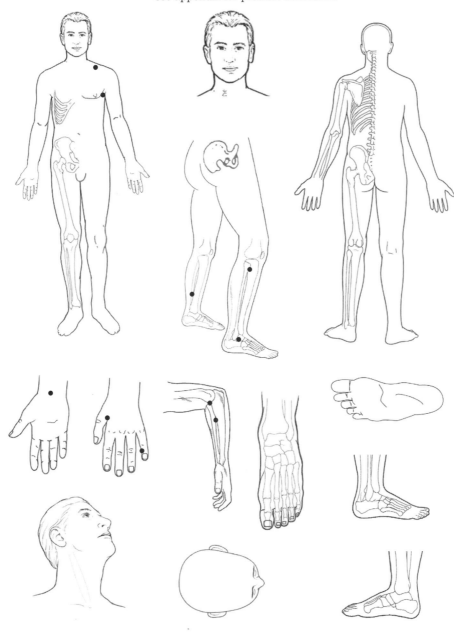

Reflex Sympathetic Dystrophy

Emergency Nutritional Daily Menu	Maintenance Nutritional Daily Menu
Glyco: 12 tsp Phyto: 2 tsp Pre-Hormone: 6 tabs Cata-Blend: 6 tabs	Glyco: 3 tsp Phyto: 2 tsp Pre-Hormone: 4 tabs Cata-Blend: 4 tabs

see appendix for product definitions

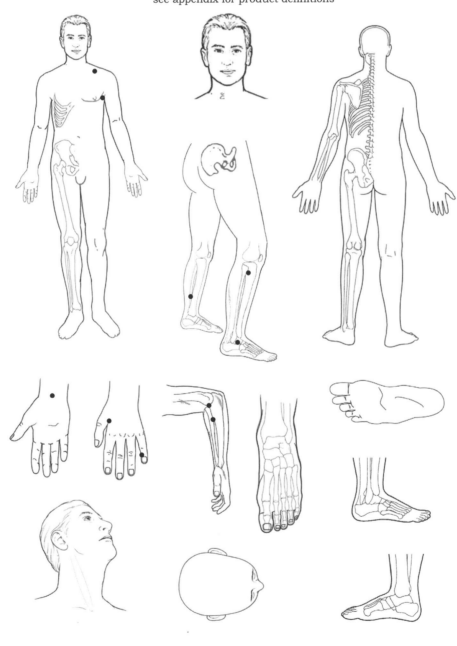

326

Renal Failure Chronic

Emergency Nutritional Daily Menu	Maintenance Nutritional Daily Menu
Glyco: 3 tsp Phyto: 1 tsp Pre-Hormone: 4 tabs Cata-Blend: 4 tabs	Glyco: 2 tsp Phyto: 1 tsp Pre-Hormone: 3 tabs Cata-Blend: 4 tabs

see appendix for product definitions

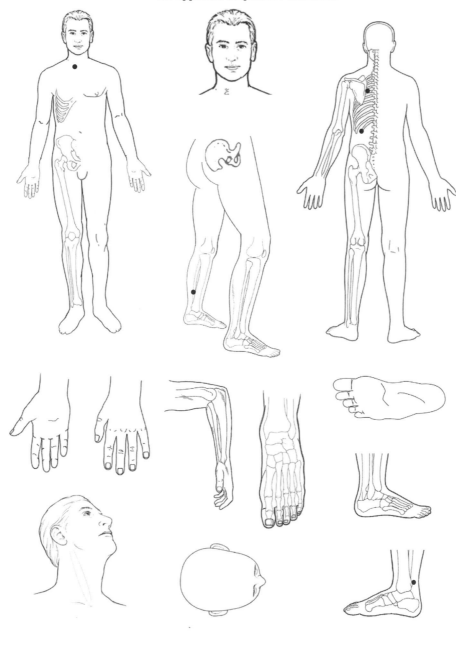

Restless Legs Syndrome

Emergency Nutritional Daily Menu	Maintenance Nutritional Daily Menu
Glyco: 3 tsp Phyto: 2 tsp Pre-Hormone: 4 tabs Cata-Blend: 4 tabs	Glyco: 1 tsp Phyto: 1 tsp Pre-Hormone: 3 tabs Cata-Blend: 4 tabs

see appendix for product definitions

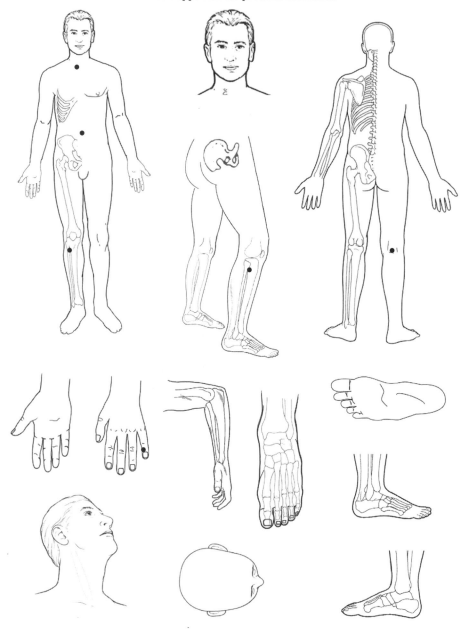

Retinitis

Emergency Nutritional Daily Menu	Maintenance Nutritional Daily Menu
Glyco: 9 tsp Phyto: 2 tsp Pre-Hormone: 4 tabs Cata-Blend: 6 tabs	Glyco: 2 tsp Phyto: 2 tsp Pre-Hormone: 3 tabs Cata-Blend: 4 tabs

see appendix for product definitions

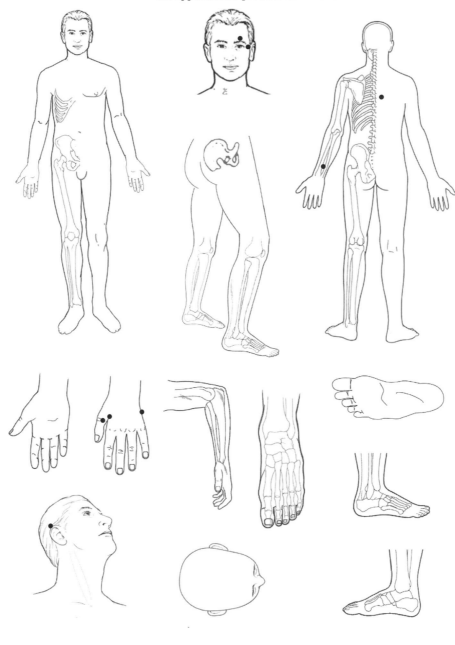

Rheumatoid Arthritis

Emergency Nutritional Daily Menu	Maintenance Nutritional Daily Menu
Glyco: 9 tsp Phyto: 2 tsp Pre-Hormone: 4 tabs Cata-Blend: 6 tabs	Glyco: 2 tsp Phyto: 2 tsp Pre-Hormone: 3 tabs Cata-Blend: 4 tabs

see appendix for product definitions

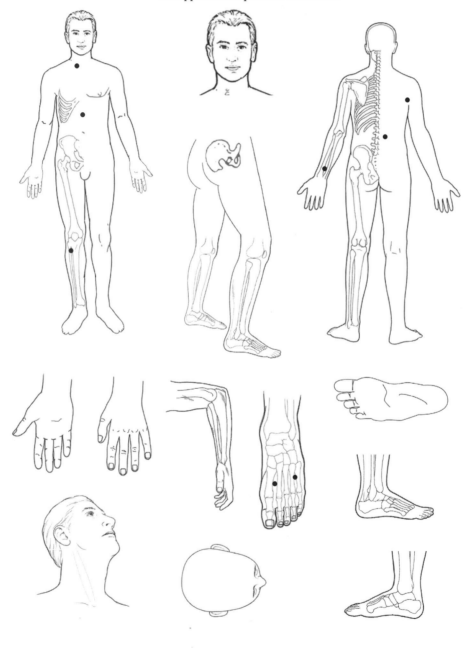

Rosacea

(apply soft laser to affect areas)

Emergency Nutritional Daily Menu	Maintenance Nutritional Daily Menu
Glyco: 3 tsp Phyto: 1/2 tsp Pre-Hormone: 4 tabs Cata-Blend: 4 tabs	Glyco: 1 tsp Phyto: 1/2 tsp Pre-Hormone: 3 tabs Cata-Blend: 4 tabs

see appendix for product definitions

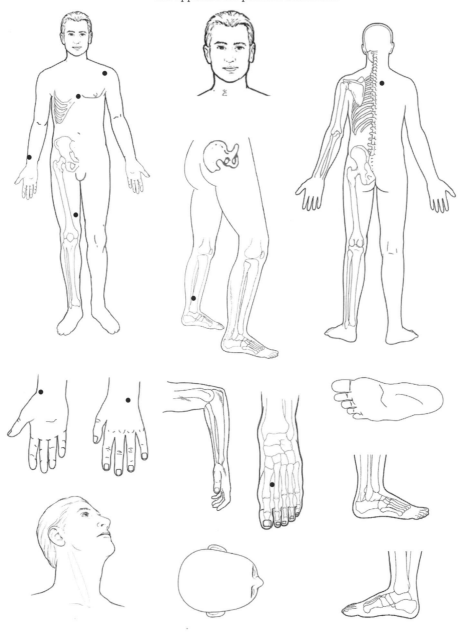

331

Sarcoidosis

Emergency Nutritional Daily Menu	Maintenance Nutritional Daily Menu
Glyco: 9 tsp Phyto: 2 tsp Pre-Hormone: 6 tabs Cata-Blend: 6 tabs	Glyco: 2 tsp Phyto: 1 tsp Pre-Hormone: 3 tabs Cata-Blend: 6 tabs

see appendix for product definitions

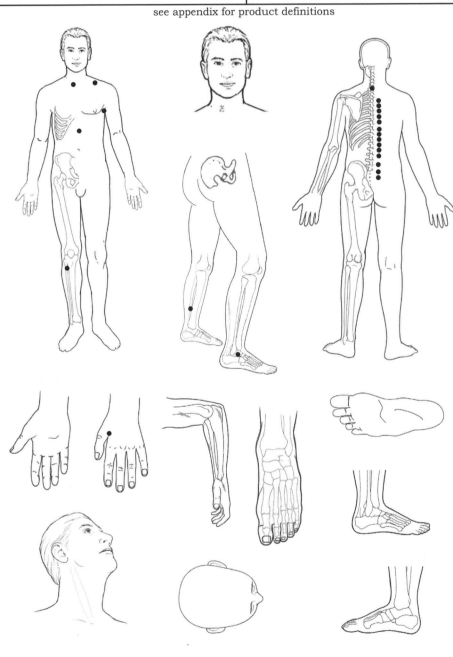

Seizure Disorder

Emergency Nutritional Daily Menu	Maintenance Nutritional Daily Menu
Glyco: 9 tsp Phyto: 1 tsp Pre-Hormone: 4 tabs Cata-Blend: 6 tabs	Glyco: 2 tsp Phyto: 1 tsp Pre-Hormone: 3 tabs Cata-Blend: 6 tabs

see appendix for product definitions

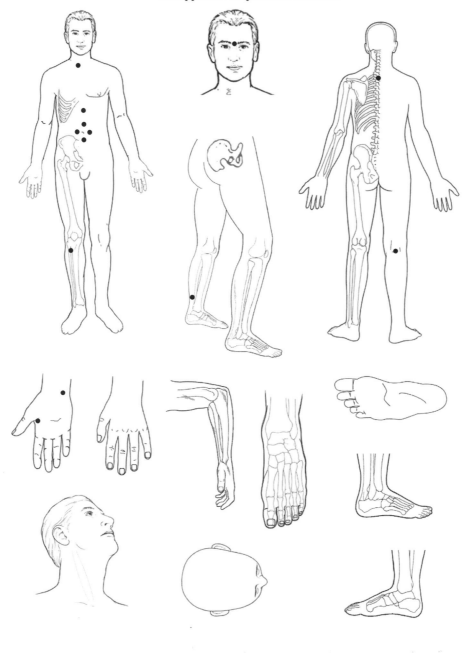

333

Sepsis

Emergency Nutritional Daily Menu	Maintenance Nutritional Daily Menu
Glyco: 15 tsp Phyto: 3 tsp Pre-Hormone: 6 tabs Cata-Blend: 6 tabs	Glyco: 3 tsp Phyto: 1 tsp Pre-Hormone: 3 tabs Cata-Blend: 6 tabs

see appendix for product definitions

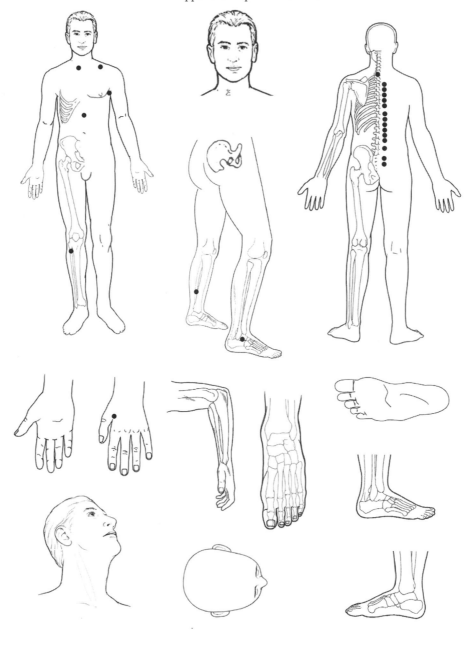

Shingles

(apply soft laser on affected areas)

Emergency Nutritional Daily Menu	Maintenance Nutritional Daily Menu
Glyco: 6 tsp Phyto: 2 tsp Pre-Hormone: 6 tabs Cata-Blend: 6 tabs	Glyco: 2 tsp Phyto: 1/2 tsp Pre-Hormone: 3 tabs Cata-Blend: 6 tabs

see appendix for product definitions

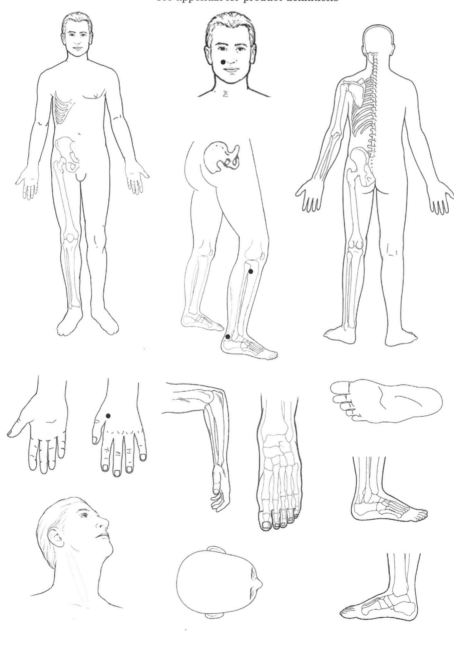

Shortness of Breath

Emergency Nutritional Daily Menu	Maintenance Nutritional Daily Menu
Glyco: 6 tsp Phyto: 1 tsp Pre-Hormone: 6 tabs Essentials: 4 tabs	Glyco: 1 tsp Phyto: 1/2 tsp Pre-Hormone: 3 tabs Essentials: 4 tabs

see appendix for product definitions

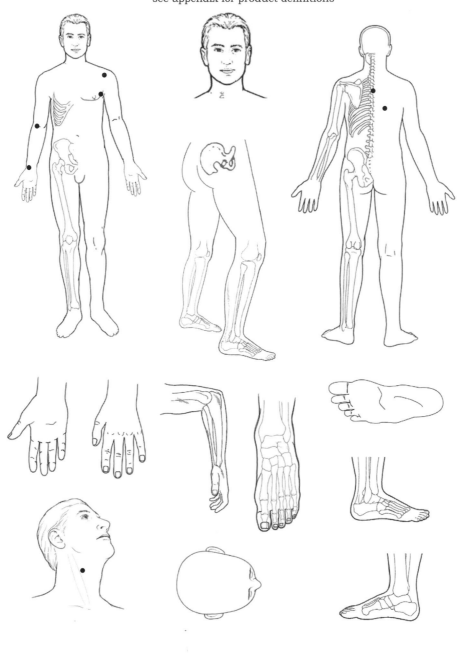

336

Sick Sinus Syndrome

Emergency Nutritional Daily Menu	Maintenance Nutritional Daily Menu
Glyco: 6 tsp Phyto: 2 tsp Pre-Hormone: 4 tabs Cata-Blend: 6 tabs	Glyco: 2 tsp Phyto: 1 tsp Pre-Hormone: 3 tabs Cata-Blend: 6 tabs

see appendix for product definitions

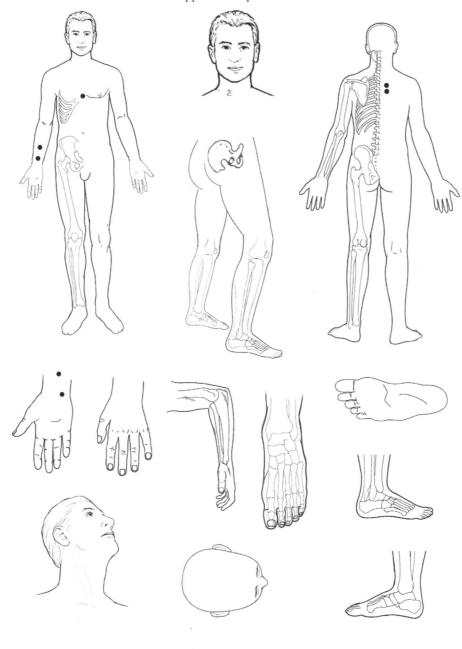

337

Sinusitis Chronic

Emergency Nutritional Daily Menu	Maintenance Nutritional Daily Menu
Glyco: 3 tsp Phyto: 2 tsp Pre-Hormone: 4 tabs Cata-Blend: 4 tabs	Glyco: 1 tsp Phyto: 1 tsp Pre-Hormone: 3 tabs Cata-Blend: 4 tabs

see appendix for product definitions

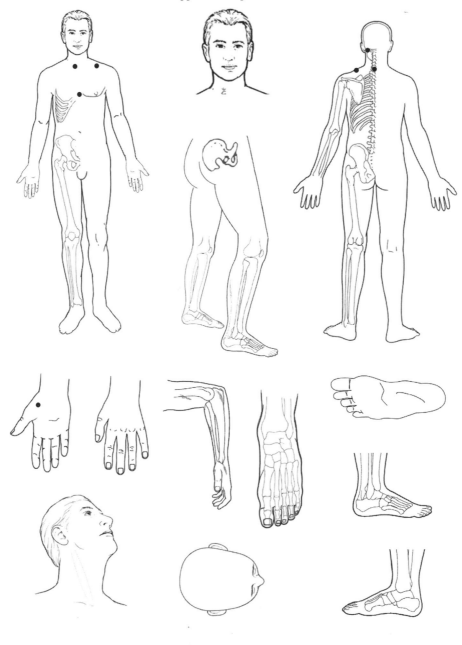

Sjogren's Syndrome

Emergency Nutritional Daily Menu	Maintenance Nutritional Daily Menu
Glyco: 9 tsp Phyto: 2 tsp Pre-Hormone: 6 tabs Cata-Blend: 6 tabs	Glyco: 2 tsp Phyto: 1 tsp Pre-Hormone: 3 tabs Cata-Blend: 6 tabs

see appendix for product definitions

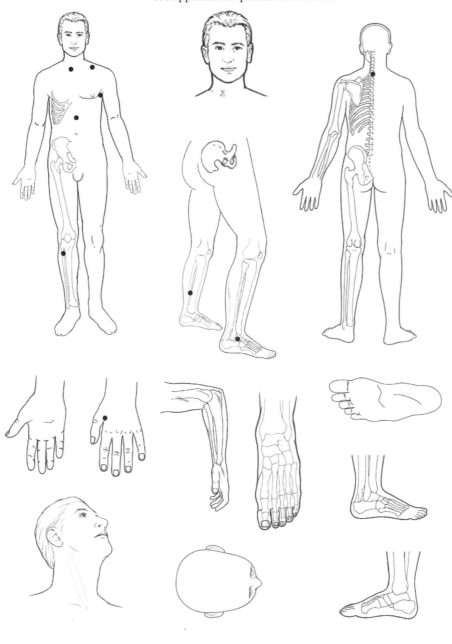

339

SLE (Systemic Lupus Erythematosis)

Emergency Nutritional Daily Menu	Maintenance Nutritional Daily Menu
Glyco: 12 tsp Phyto: 2 tsp Pre-Hormone: 6 tabs Cata-Blend: 6 tabs	Glyco: 2 tsp Phyto: 1 tsp Pre-Hormone: 4 tabs Cata-Blend: 6 tabs

see appendix for product definitions

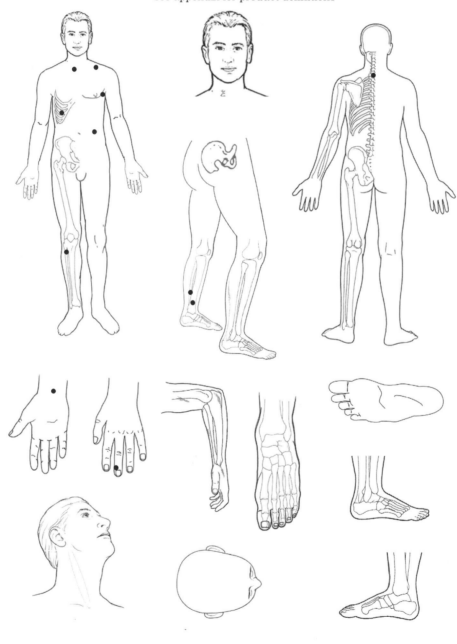

Sleep Apnea

Emergency Nutritional Daily Menu	Maintenance Nutritional Daily Menu
Glyco: 3 tsp Phyto: 1 tsp Pre-Hormone: 4 tabs Cata-Blend: 4 tabs	Glyco: 1 tsp Phyto: 1 tsp Pre-Hormone: 3 tabs Cata-Blend: 4 tabs

see appendix for product definitions

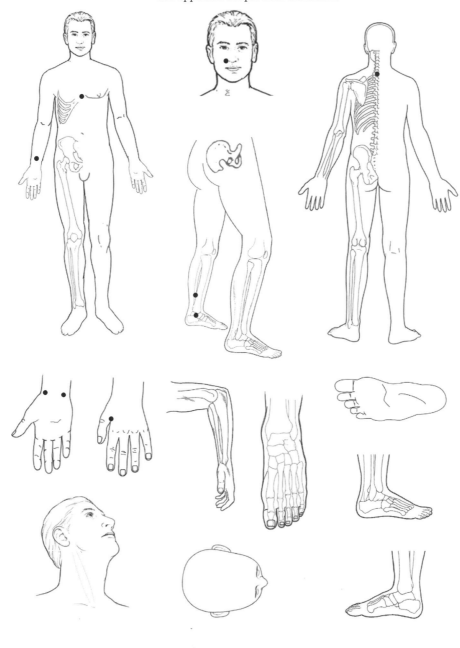

Smallpox

Emergency Nutritional Daily Menu	Maintenance Nutritional Daily Menu
Glyco: 12 tsp Phyto: 2 tsp Pre-Hormone: 6 tabs Cata-Blend: 6 tabs	Glyco: 2 tsp Phyto: 1 tsp Pre-Hormone: 3 tabs Cata-Blend: 6 tabs

see appendix for product definitions

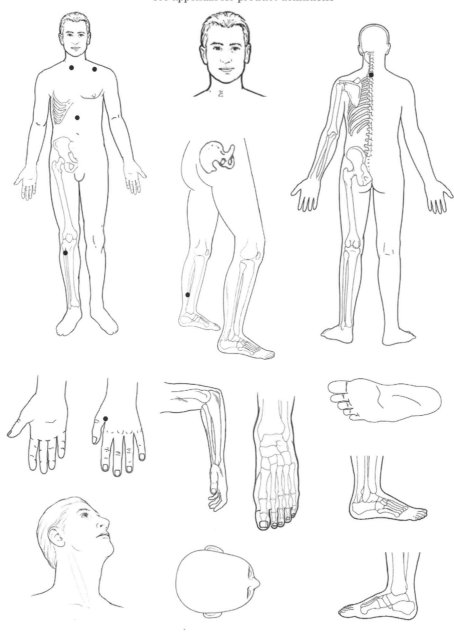

342

Sore Throat

Emergency Nutritional Daily Menu	Maintenance Nutritional Daily Menu
Glyco: 3 tsp Phyto: 1 tsp Pre-Hormone: 4 tabs Essentials: 4 tabs	Glyco: 1/2 tsp Phyto: 1/2 tsp Pre-Hormone: 3 tabs Essentials: 4 tabs

see appendix for product definitions

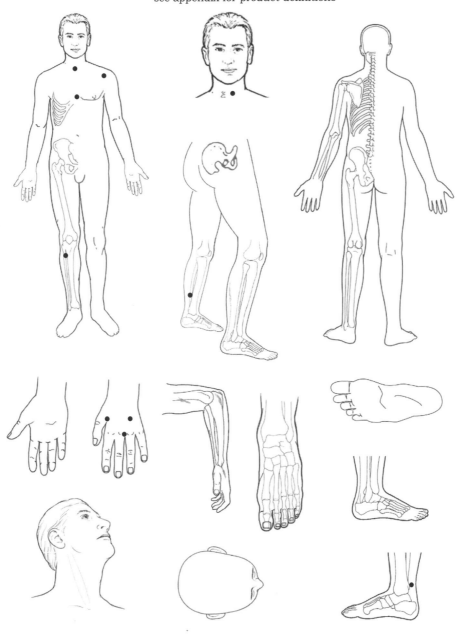

343

Spleen Infection

Emergency Nutritional Daily Menu	Maintenance Nutritional Daily Menu
Glyco: 6 tsp Phyto: 2 tsp Pre-Hormone: 6 tabs Essentials: 4 tabs	Glyco: 1 tsp Phyto: 1 tsp Pre-Hormone: 3 tabs Essentials: 4 tabs

see appendix for product definitions

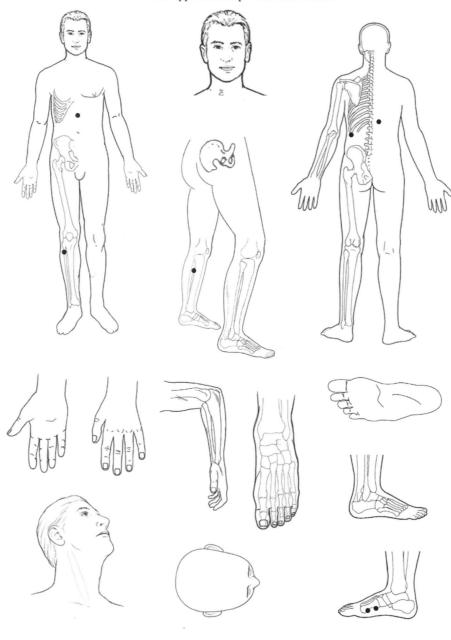

Splenomegaly

Emergency Nutritional Daily Menu	Maintenance Nutritional Daily Menu
Glyco: 6 tsp Phyto: 1 tsp Pre-Hormone: 4 tabs Essentials: 4 tabs	Glyco: 1 tsp Phyto: 1/2 tsp Pre-Hormone: 3 tabs Essentials: 4 tabs

see appendix for product definitions

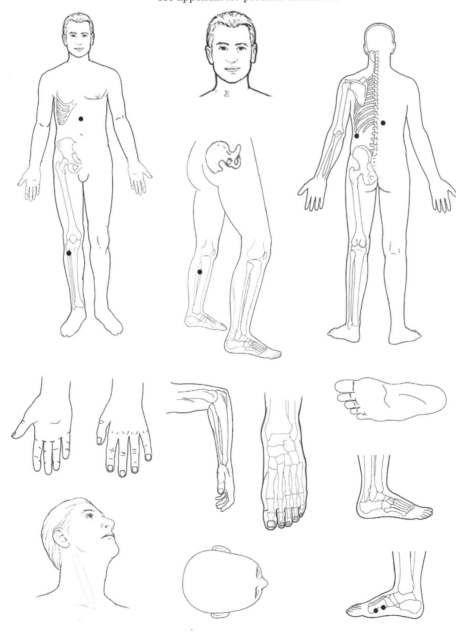

Staphylococcal Food Poisoning (Detoxification)

Emergency Nutritional Daily Menu	Maintenance Nutritional Daily Menu
Glyco: 6 tsp Phyto: 1 tsp Pre-Hormone: 4 tabs Essentials: 4 tabs	Glyco: 1/2 tsp Phyto: 1/2 tsp Pre-Hormone: 3 tabs Essentials: 4 tabs

see appendix for product definitions

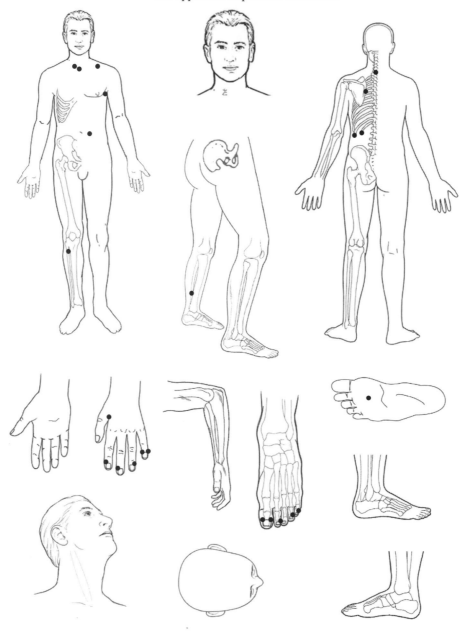

346

Stomach Problems

Emergency Nutritional Daily Menu	Maintenance Nutritional Daily Menu
Glyco: 6 tsp Phyto: 1 tsp Pre-Hormone: 4 tabs Essentials: 4 tabs	Glyco: 1 tsp Phyto: 1/2 tsp Pre-Hormone: 3 tabs Essentials: 4 tabs

see appendix for product definitions

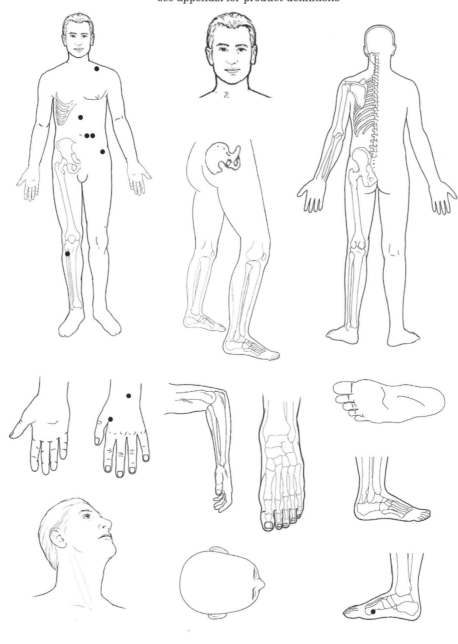

Stomatitis

Emergency Nutritional Daily Menu	Maintenance Nutritional Daily Menu
Glyco: 6 tsp Phyto: 1 tsp Pre-Hormone: 4 tabs Essentials: 4 tabs	Glyco: 1/2 tsp Phyto: 1/2 tsp Pre-Hormone: 3 tabs Essentials: 4 tabs

see appendix for product definitions

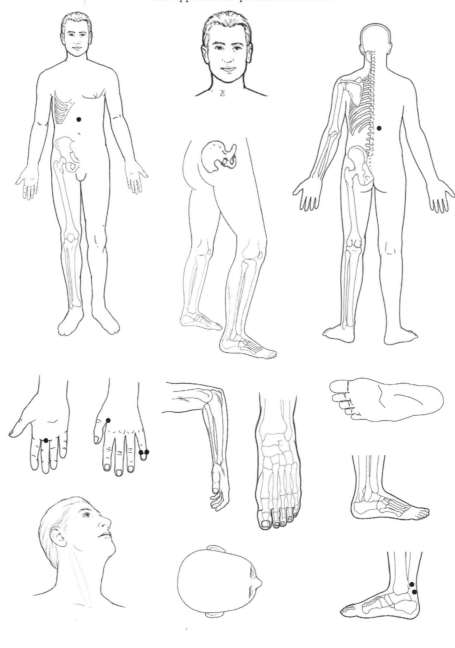

348

Strep Throat (Pharyngitis)

Emergency Nutritional Daily Menu	Maintenance Nutritional Daily Menu
Glyco: 6 tsp Phyto: 2 tsp Pre-Hormone: 4 tabs Essentials: 4 tabs	Glyco: 1/2 tsp Phyto: 1/2 tsp Pre-Hormone: 3 tabs Essentials: 4 tabs

see appendix for product definitions

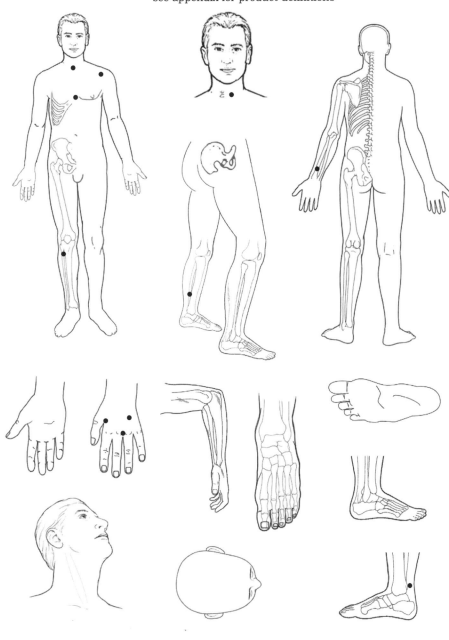

Stress (Physical or Emotional)

Emergency Nutritional Daily Menu	Maintenance Nutritional Daily Menu
Glyco: 6 tsp Phyto: 2 tsp Pre-Hormone: 6 tabs Essentials: 4 tabs	Glyco: 1 tsp Phyto: 1/2 tsp Pre-Hormone: 3 tabs Essentials: 4 tabs

see appendix for product definitions

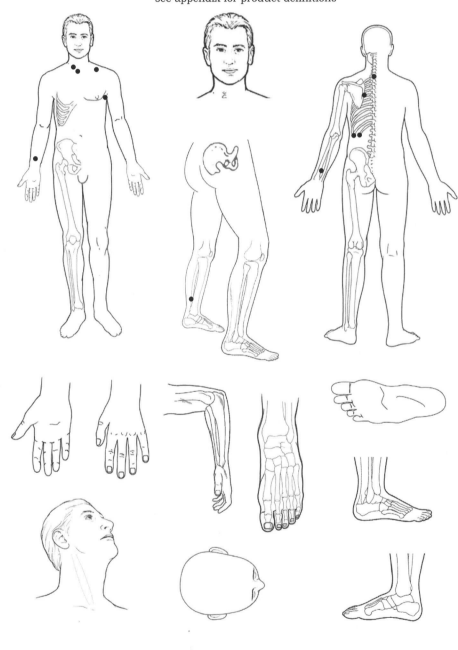

Sugar Craving

Emergency Nutritional Daily Menu	Maintenance Nutritional Daily Menu
Glyco: 6 tsp Phyto: 1 tsp Pre-Hormone: 6 tabs Cata-Blend: 4 tabs	Glyco: 1 tsp Phyto: 1/2 tsp Pre-Hormone: 3 tabs Cata-Blend: 4 tabs

see appendix for product definitions

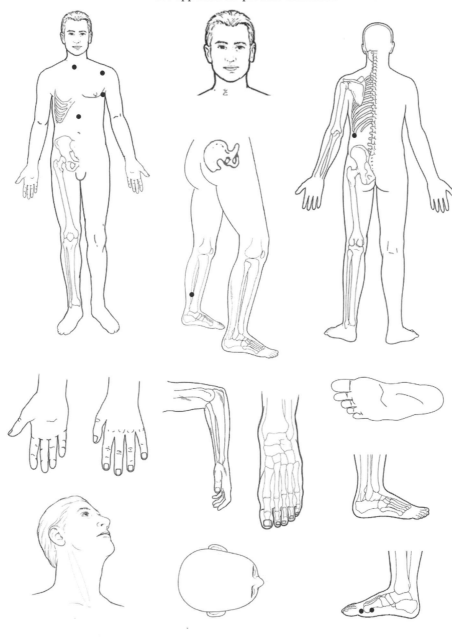

Surgery (During Recovery)

Emergency Nutritional Daily Menu	Maintenance Nutritional Daily Menu
Glyco: 6 tsp Phyto: 2 tsp Pre-Hormone: 6 tabs Cata-Blend: 6 tabs	Glyco: NA Phyto: NA Pre-Hormone: 3 tabs Cata-Blend: 6 tabs

see appendix for product definitions

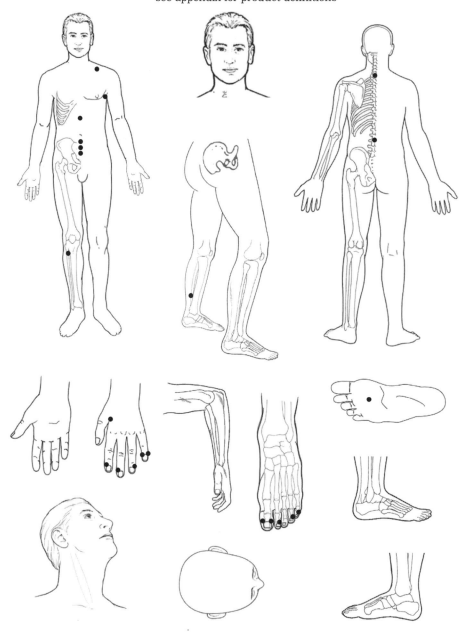

Systemic Lupus Erythematosis (SLE)

Emergency Nutritional Daily Menu	Maintenance Nutritional Daily Menu
Glyco: 12 tsp Phyto: 2 tsp Pre-Hormone: 6 tabs Cata-Blend: 6 tabs	Glyco: 2 tsp Phyto: 1 tsp Pre-Hormone: 4 tabs Cata-Blend: 6 tabs

see appendix for product definitions

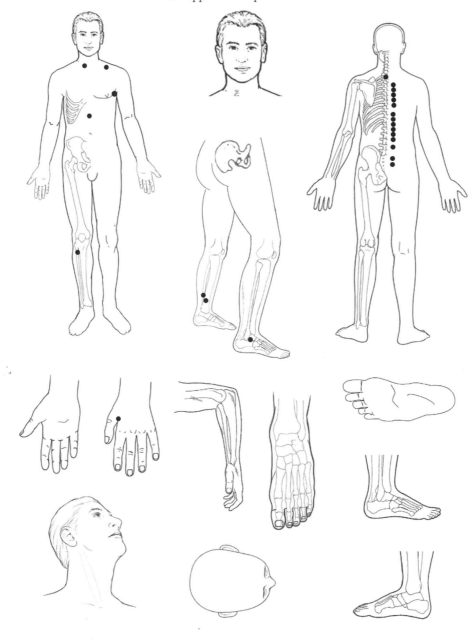

Temporal Arteritis

Emergency Nutritional Daily Menu	Maintenance Nutritional Daily Menu
Glyco: 12 tsp Phyto: 3 tsp Pre-Hormone: 6 tabs Cata-Blend: 6 tabs	Glyco: 2 tsp Phyto: 1 tsp Pre-Hormone: 3 tabs Cata-Blend: 6 tabs

see appendix for product definitions

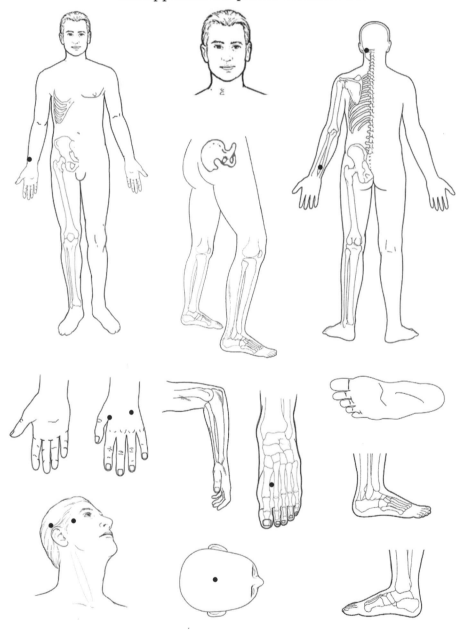

Tension Headache (Chronic)

Emergency Nutritional Daily Menu	Maintenance Nutritional Daily Menu
Glyco: 3 tsp Phyto: 1 tsp Pre-Hormone: 4 tabs Cata-Blend: 4 tabs	Glyco: 1 tsp Phyto: 1/2 tsp Pre-Hormone: 4 tabs Cata-Blend: 4 tabs

see appendix for product definitions

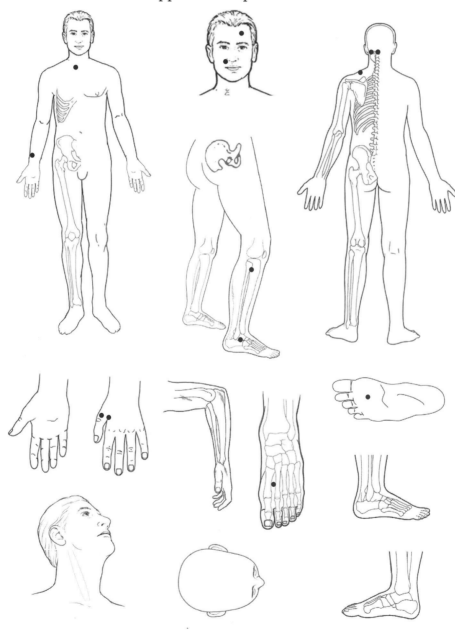

355

Thrombocytopenia

Emergency Nutritional Daily Menu	Maintenance Nutritional Daily Menu
Glyco: 6 tsp Phyto: 1 tsp Pre-Hormone: 4 tabs Cata-Blend: 4 tabs	Glyco: 1 tsp Phyto: 1/2 tsp Pre-Hormone: 3 tabs Cata-Blend: 4 tabs

see appendix for product definitions

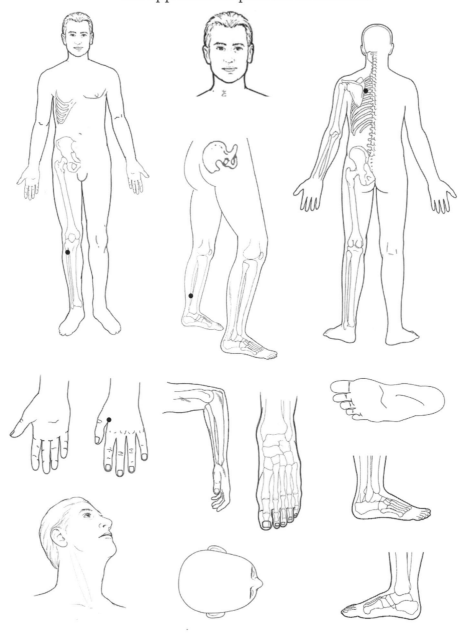

Thyroiditis (Acute)

Emergency Nutritional Daily Menu	Maintenance Nutritional Daily Menu
Glyco: 12 tsp Phyto: 1 tsp Pre-Hormone: 4 tabs Cata-Blend: 6 tabs	Glyco: 1 tsp Phyto: 1/2 tsp Pre-Hormone: 3 tabs Cata-Blend: 6 tabs

see appendix for product definitions

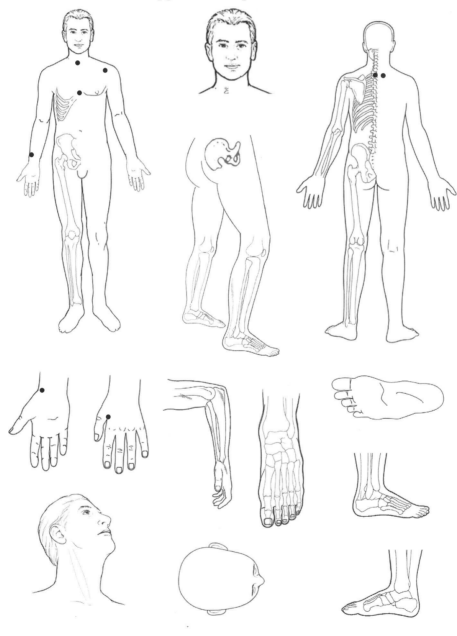

Tissue Trauma

Emergency Nutritional Daily Menu	Maintenance Nutritional Daily Menu
Glyco: 12 tsp Phyto: 3 tsp Pre-Hormone: 6 tabs Cata-Blend: 6 tabs	Glyco: 2 tsp Phyto: 1 tsp Pre-Hormone: 3 tabs Cata-Blend: 6 tabs

see appendix for product definitions

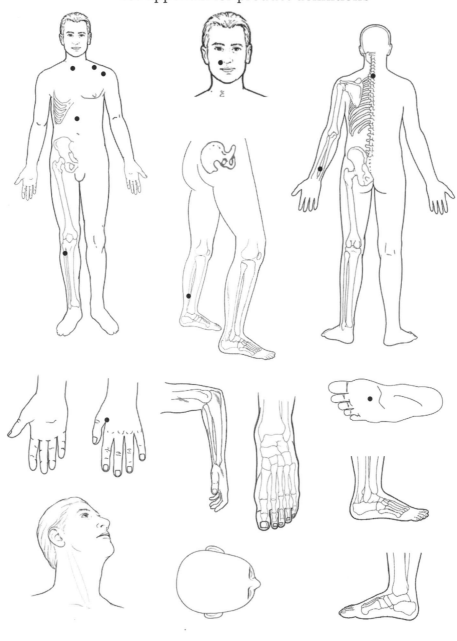

Tobacco Dependence

Emergency Nutritional Daily Menu	Maintenance Nutritional Daily Menu
Glyco: 3 tsp Phyto: 1 tsp Pre-Hormone: 4 tabs Cata-Blend: 4 tabs	Glyco: 1 tsp Phyto: 1 tsp Pre-Hormone: 3 tabs Cata-Blend: 4 tabs

see appendix for product definitions

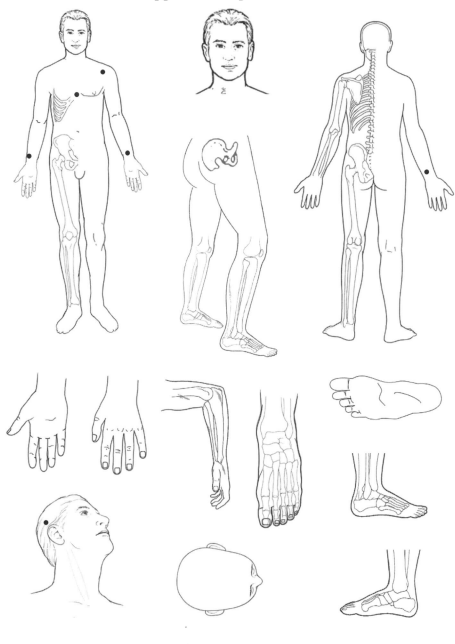

Tonsillitis

Emergency Nutritional Daily Menu	Maintenance Nutritional Daily Menu
Glyco: 3 tsp Phyto: 1 tsp Pre-Hormone: 4 tabs Essentials: 4 tabs	Glyco: 1/2 tsp Phyto: 1/2 tsp Pre-Hormone: 3 tabs Essentials: 4 tabs

see appendix for product definitions

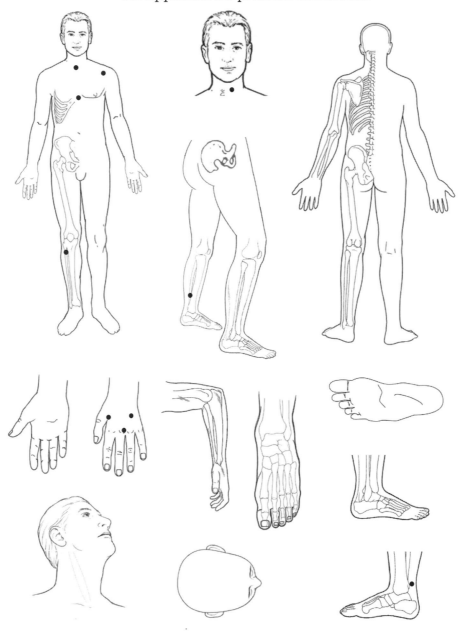

Tonsils (Swollen)

Emergency Nutritional Daily Menu	Maintenance Nutritional Daily Menu
Glyco: 3 tsp Phyto: 1 tsp Pre-Hormone: 4 tabs Essentials: 4 tabs	Glyco: 1/2 tsp Phyto: 1/2 tsp Pre-Hormone: 3 tabs Essentials: 4 tabs

see appendix for product definitions

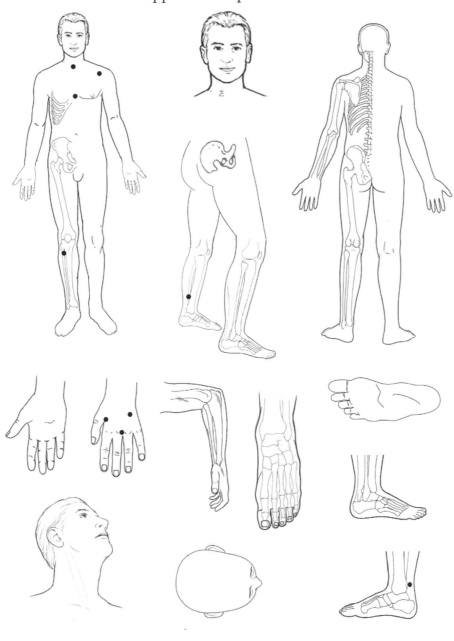

Ulcerative Colitis

Emergency Nutritional Daily Menu	Maintenance Nutritional Daily Menu
Glyco: 9 tsp Phyto: 2 tsp Pre-Hormone: 4 tabs Cata-Blend: 6 tabs	Glyco: 2 tsp Phyto: 1 tsp Pre-Hormone: 3 tabs Cata-Blend: 6 tabs

see appendix for product definitions

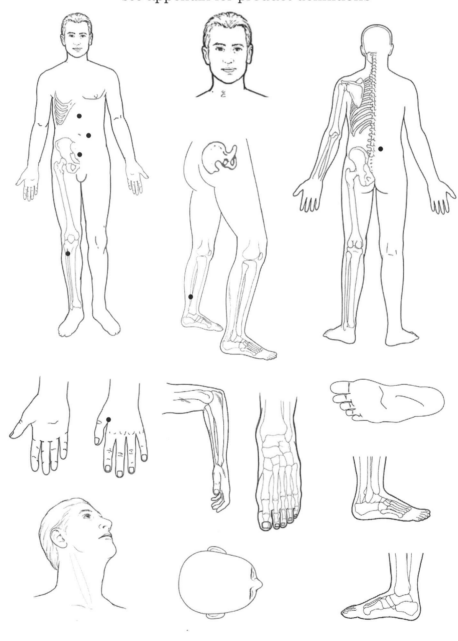

Ulcers- Diabetic

(soft laser over affected area)

Emergency Nutritional Daily Menu	Maintenance Nutritional Daily Menu
Glyco: 4 tsp Phyto: 3 tsp Pre-Hormone: 6 tabs Cata-Blend: 6 tabs	Glyco: 2 tsp Phyto: 2 tsp Pre-Hormone: 4 tabs Cata-Blend: 6 tabs

see appendix for product definitions

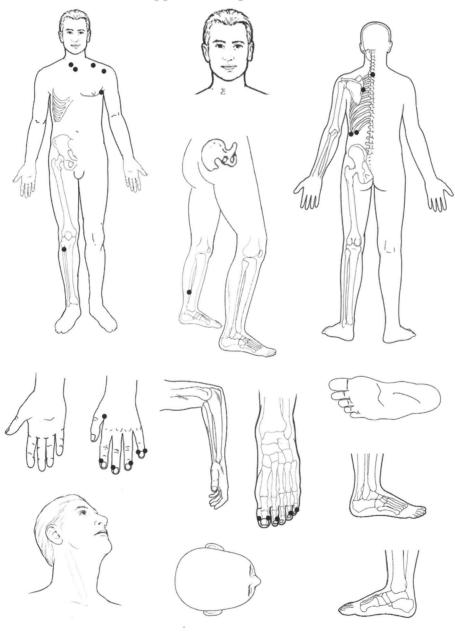

Urethritis

Emergency Nutritional Daily Menu	Maintenance Nutritional Daily Menu
Glyco: 3 tsp Phyto: 1 tsp Pre-Hormone: 4 tabs Essentials: 4 tabs	Glyco: 1 tsp Phyto: 1/2 tsp Pre-Hormone: 3 tabs Essentials: 4 tabs

see appendix for product definitions

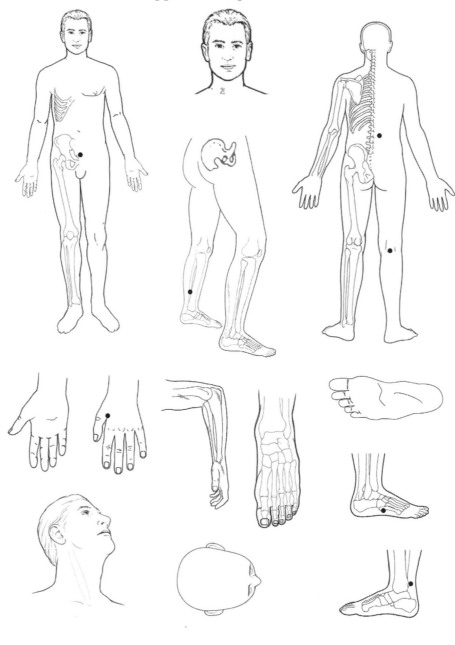

Urinary Tract Infection (UTI)

Emergency Nutritional Daily Menu	Maintenance Nutritional Daily Menu
Glyco: 3 tsp Phyto: 1 tsp Pre-Hormone: 4 tabs Essentials: 4 tabs	Glyco: 1 tsp Phyto: 1/2 tsp Pre-Hormone: 3 tabs Essentials: 4 tabs

see appendix for product definitions

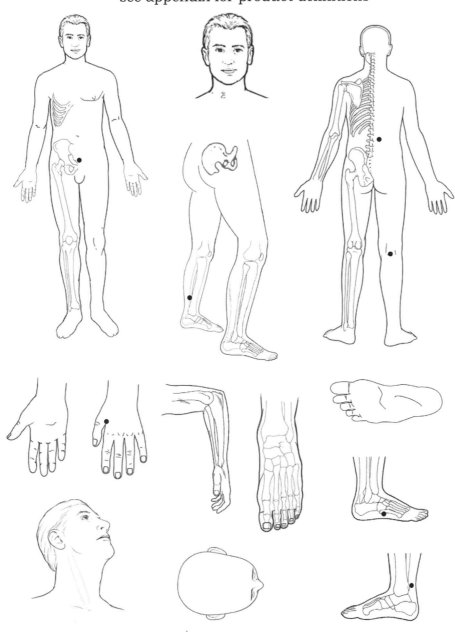

Uterine Fibroids

Emergency Nutritional Daily Menu	Maintenance Nutritional Daily Menu
Glyco: 3 tsp Phyto: 1 tsp Pre-Hormone: 4 tabs Essentials: 4 tabs	Glyco: 1 tsp Phyto: 1/2 tsp Pre-Hormone: 3 tabs Essentials: 4 tabs

see appendix for product definitions

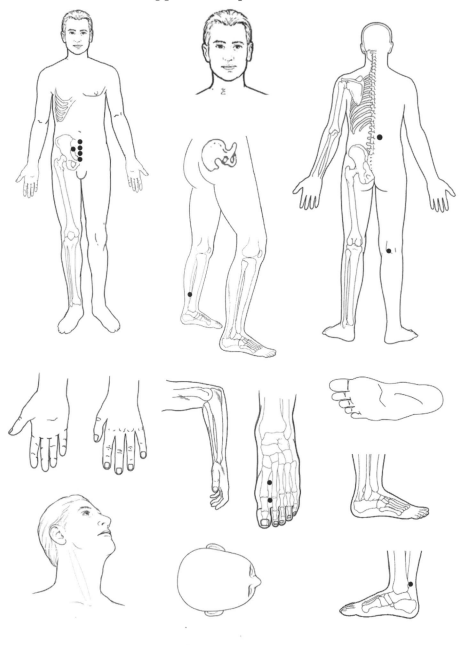

Vaginitis/Vulvitis (Candida)

Emergency Nutritional Daily Menu	Maintenance Nutritional Daily Menu
Glyco: 3 tsp Phyto: 2 tsp Pre-Hormone: 4 tabs Essentials: 4 tabs	Glyco: 1 tsp Phyto: 1/2 tsp Pre-Hormone: 3 tabs Essentials: 4 tabs

see appendix for product definitions

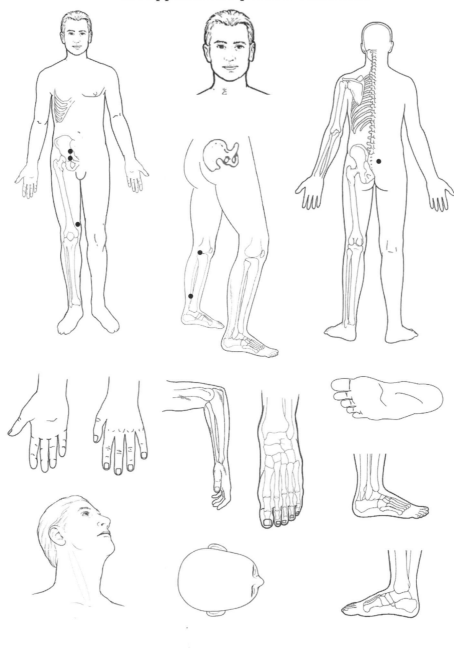

Varicella (Chickenpox)

Emergency Nutritional Daily Menu	Maintenance Nutritional Daily Menu
Glyco: 6 tsp Phyto: 2 tsp Pre-Hormone: 3 tabs Essentials: 4 tabs	Glyco: 1/2 tsp Phyto: 1/2 tsp Pre-Hormone: 3 tabs Essentials: 4 tabs

see appendix for product definitions

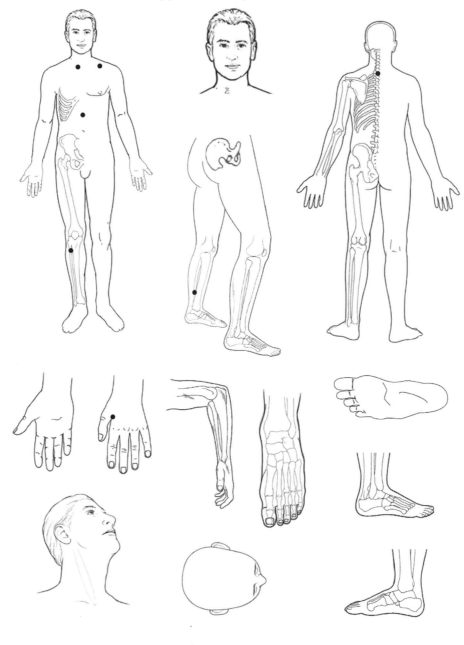

Vasculitis

Emergency Nutritional Daily Menu	Maintenance Nutritional Daily Menu
Glyco: 12 tsp Phyto: 2 tsp Pre-Hormone: 6 tabs Cata-Blend: 6 tabs	Glyco: 2 tsp Phyto: 1 tsp Pre-Hormone: 3 tabs Cata-Blend: 6 tabs

see appendix for product definitions

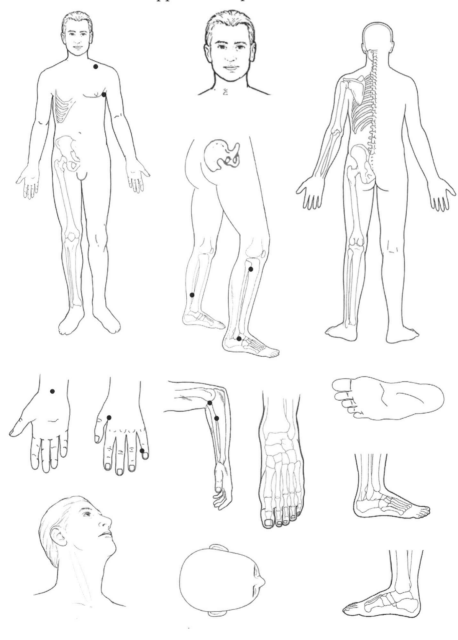

Venereal Disease

Emergency Nutritional Daily Menu	Maintenance Nutritional Daily Menu
Glyco: 9 tsp Phyto: 2 tsp Pre-Hormone: 3 tabs Essentials: 4 tabs	Glyco: 1 tsp Phyto: 1 tsp Pre-Hormone: 3 tabs Essentials: 4 tabs

see appendix for product definitions

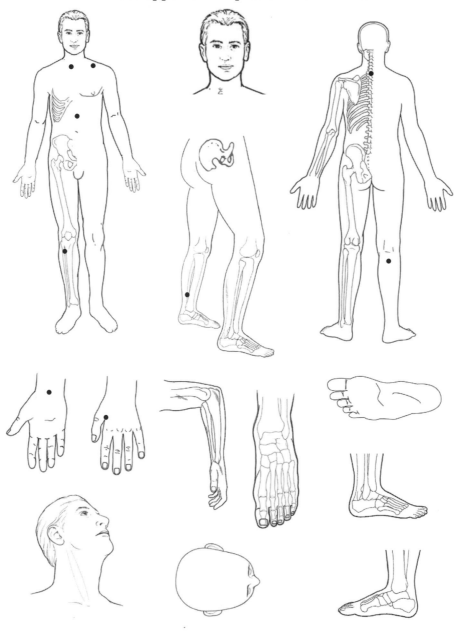

Vertigo (Dizziness)

Emergency Nutritional Daily Menu	Maintenance Nutritional Daily Menu
Glyco: 9 tsp Phyto: 2 tsp Pre-Hormone: 4 tabs Essentials: 4 tabs	Glyco: 1 tsp Phyto: 1/2 tsp Pre-Hormone: 3 tabs Essentials: 4 tabs

see appendix for product definitions

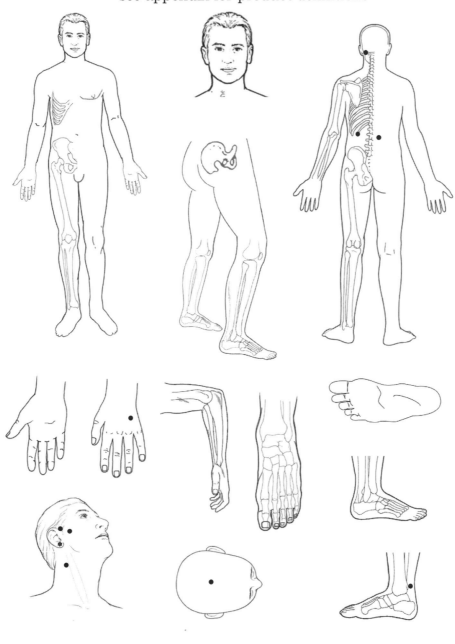

Viral Infection

Emergency Nutritional Daily Menu	Maintenance Nutritional Daily Menu
Glyco: 6 tsp Phyto: 2 tsp Pre-Hormone: 4 tabs Cata-Blend: 4 tabs	Glyco: 1 tsp Phyto: 1 tsp Pre-Hormone: 3 tabs Cata-Blend: 4 tabs

see appendix for product definitions

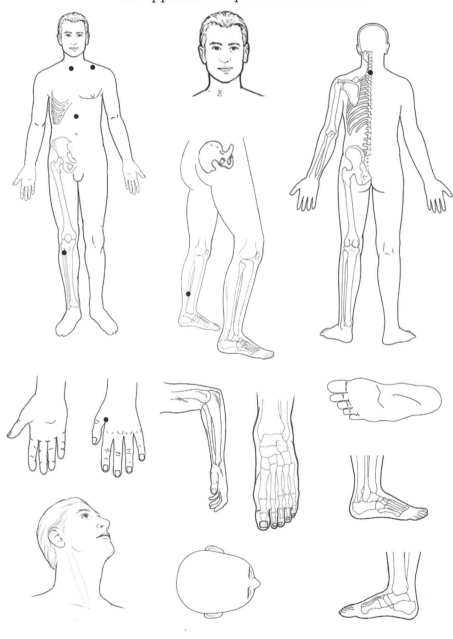

Warts

Emergency Nutritional Daily Menu	Maintenance Nutritional Daily Menu
Glyco: 6 tsp Phyto: 2 tsp Pre-Hormone: 4 tabs Essentials: 4 tabs	Glyco: 1/2 tsp Phyto: 1/2 tsp Pre-Hormone: 3 tabs Essentials: 4 tabs

see appendix for product definitions

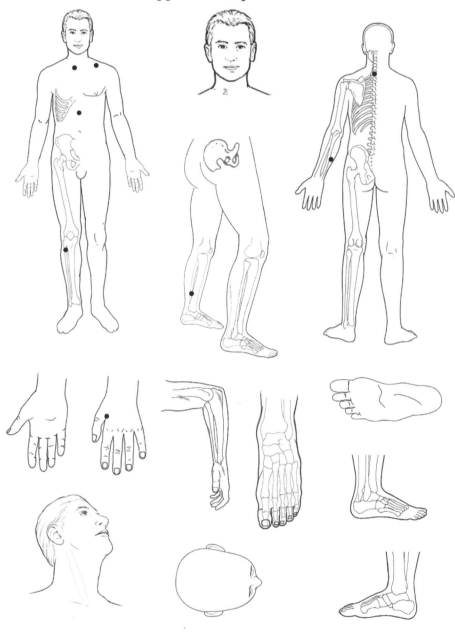

"He who cures a disease may be the skillfullest, but he that prevents it is the safest physician."
-T. Fuller

PART III:
Recommendations for Conditions Not Listed

375

"I have a right to decide what happens to my own body, not because I know more than anybody else, but simply because it is my body. And I have a right to acquire the information that can help me make those crucial decisions."
-A. Lorde

Recommendations for Conditions Not Listed

Glyco = Glyconutrients (monosaccharides)
Maintenance*: 1 capsule 3 times a day (1/4 tsp 1 or 2 x day).
Medical Challenge*: 1 tsp. 2 times a day (6 caps 4 x day)
Severe Medical Challenge*: 4teaspoons to 6 tablespoons 4 x day

Phyto = Phytochemicals (antioxidants)
Maintenance*: 1 capsule 2 times a day (1/2 tsp day)
Medical Challenge*: 2 caps 3x day or 1/2 tsp 3 x a day
Severe Medical Challenge*: 2 to 4 teaspoons 2 times a day

Pre-Hormone: Beta Sitosterol Complex (Mexican yam)
Maintenance*: 1 capsule 3 times a day.
Medical Challenge*: Serving Size: 2 capsules 3 times a day
Severe Medical Challenge*: 3 capsules 3 times a day

Essentials - Complete Minerals and Vitamins and Antioxidants
Maintenance*: 2 capsules 2 times a day
Medical Challenge*: 2 capsules 3 times day
Severe Medical Challenge*: 2 capsules 3 times a day

Catablend - Complete Minerals and Vitamins with extra Antioxidants
Maintenance*: 2 capsules 2 times a day
Medical Challenge*: 2 capsules 3 times day
Severe Medical Challenge*: 2 capsules 3 times a day

Key to Terms
*Maintenance: Prevention
*Medical Challenge: illness now or illness in the past; not an immediate threat to life
*Severe Medical Challenge: illness leading to severe compromise life

See Appendix for Product Definitions

377

"The superior doctor prevents sickness;
The mediocre doctor attends to impending sickness;
The inferior doctor treats actual sickness."
-Chinese Proverb

378

PART IV: Appendix

379

"What lies behind us and what lies before us
are tiny matters compared to what lies within us."
-Emerson

Appendix 1

Product Definitions Nutritional Daily Menu

Glyco:
Ambrotose™
Company: Mannatech, Inc.
www.mannatech.com
Phone: see local directory

Phyto:
Phytaloe®
Company: Mannatech, Inc.
www.mannatech.com
Phone: see local directory

Pre-Hormone:
Plus
Company: Mannatech, Inc.
www.mannatech.com
Phone: see local directory

Essentials
Glycentials™
Company: Mannatech, Inc.
www.mannatech.com
Phone: see local directory

Cata-Blend:
Catalyst™
Company: Mannatech, Inc.
www.mannatech.com
Phone: see local directory

RESOURCES

ORGANIC CONSUMERS ASSOCIATION

An online resource for listings of where to find organic retailers in your area. Also contains a multitude of information and the latest news regarding organic standards, genetically engineered foods, rBHT, Mad Cow Disease, irradiation and food safety.

www.organicconsumers.org

COALITION FOR NATURAL HEALTH

Their mission is to protect every citizen's right to natural health freedom of choice. This includes the practitioner's right to practice and the consumer's right to access natural health options. CNH actively opposes legislation that would restrict or revoke a practitioner's right to provide consultation and make recommendations aimed at educating the consumer about natural health-related techniques and choices that promote a healthier lifestyle. CNH actively supports legislation that protects rights of natural healers and practitioners of holistic health modalities to practice. CNH also diligently attempts to educate consumers and legislators alike, regarding the role of natural health modalities in promoting wellness.

www.naturalhealth.org

Test Your Drinking Water
American Environmental Health Foundation
8345 Walnut Hill Ln
Dallas, TX 75231
Phone: 1-800-428-2343

www.ehcd.com

Spring Water (glass bottles) Mountain Valley
Mountain Valley Spring Co.
PO Box 1610
Hot Spr. National Park
AR 71902
Phone: 1-800-643-1501

www.mountainvalleyspring.com

Natural Lifestyle A wonderful resource for a variety of organic foods, natural cookware, cleaning products, organic cotton clothing, teas and more. Order their catalogue by mail – it is easier to see all of their products than on their website.

16 Lookout Drive
Asheville, NC 28804-3330
Phone: 1-800-752-2775

www.natural-lifestyle.com

Eat Wild A source to learn more about grass-fed beef and even find a local producer.

www.eatwild.com

Mac Nut Oil is a healthy, monounsaturated oil that is wonderful on salads, and because it can withstand high temperatures without developing dangerous trans fatty acids, it can even be used for cooking. It is a nutritious and delicious alternative to other oils.

PO Box 864066
Plano, TX 75086-4066
Phone: 1-866-462-2688

www.macnutoil.com

ORGANIC HERBS, SEASONINGS, FACIAL PRODUCTS

Mountain Rose Herbs Online source for many herbs like Red Clover, Uva Ursi, Black Cohosh, Chaste Tree Berry; as well as herbal seasonings; face and body products; woman's products; bulk cosmetic ingredients like clay, beeswax or vegetable glycerin and even glass jars for storing your homemade beauty products.

85472 Dilley Lane
Eugene, OR 97405
Phone: 1-541-741-7341
Phone: 1-800-879-3337
Fax: 1-510-217-4012
e-mail: info@mountainroseherbs.com

www.mountainroseherbs.com

ORGANIC COTTON AND FEMALE PRODUCTS

Natracare Organic 100% cotton feminine care products.

Phone: 1-303-617-3476
Fax: 1-303-617-3495

www.natracare.com

Organic Essentials Source for organic cotton products including cotton balls, swabs and nursing pads.

822 Baldridge Street
O'Donnell, Texas 79351
Phone: 1-806-428-3486
Fax: 1-806-428-3475

www.organicessentials.com

HORMONE TESTING

NRG Solutions is a company that can send you a test that measures hormone levels over a 24-hour period through your saliva. The test is done at home and does not require a prescription or doctor's order. After obtaining your results, you can work with your physician to find a plant-based source of natural hormone replacement, or obtain a standard hormonal cream directly from NRG. In addition, NRG is able to custom blend a formula specifically for you based upon your lab results. That means that your hormone treatment cream will be formulated purposely for your unique hormonal responses and needs.

7337 Canterbury Place
Downers Grove, IL, 60516
Phone: 1-630-853-8383

www.nrgsolutions.net

HEALING SUPPLIES

Marmapoint offers a full range of physician recommended products to support the healing process in an office, hospital or home setting. Included are soft lasers and teisheins for meridian point and scar tissue stimulation. Product line also includes Qi Gong machine, Guasha tools, Five-Element Music and Homeopathy.

www.marmapoint.com

FULL SPECTRUM LIGHTS

Bio-Light Group Apply the therapeutic benefits of sunlight indoors. These full spectrum lights simulate natural sunlight. Highly recommended for hospitalized patients or those bedridden or confined to indoor environment for an extended period of time.

Biologically beneficial lighting pioneers
Phone: 1-800-234-3724; 805-564-3467
Fax: 1-805-564-2147

www.biolightgroup.com

NATURAL COSMETICS AND SKIN CARE

Dr. Hauschka Highly recommended natural skin care and cosmetic company. Their products contain no chemical preservatives.

59C North Street
Hatfield, MA 01038
Phone: 1-800-247-9907
Fax: 1-413-247-5633

www.drhauschka.com

Beeswork A great source of natural face, body and bath products, as well as lip balm and candles.

122 Hamilton Drive, Suite D
Novato, Ca 94949
Phone: 1-415-883-5660
Fax: 1-415-883-6038

www.beeswork.com

SUPPLEMENTS

Carlson Laboratories Source of Vitamin E (ask for E-Gems Elite), Fish Oil and Cod Liver Oil.

Phone: 888-234-5656

www.carlsonlabs.com

Standard Process Whole food nutritional supplements made from organic foods. Standard Process products are available through qualified health professionals only.

www.standardprocess.com

Flower Essences

Bach Flower Essences are gentle homeopathic remedies that work in conjunction with any other healing modality without interaction or side effects. Many health care practitioners including naturopaths, chiropractors, dentists, and other alternative healers use them. They work by energetically helping to improve our coping mechanisms to reduce stress, alleviate worry and anxiety, and feel an increased sense of well-being.

100 Research Drive
Wilmington, MA 01887
Phone:1-800-319-9191
      1-800-338-0843
      1-978-988-3833

www.nelsonbach.com

Organic Teas

St. Dalfour Organic Teas offers certified organic black and green teas in bags. In addition to Classic Breakfast and Earl Grey teas, they have a wide range of flavored teas. Flavors include: Golden Peach, Lemon tea, Strawberry, Black Cherry, Peppermint, Cinnamon Apple Green, Golden Mango Green, Ginger Honey Green, Strawberry Rose Green, Mandarin Orange Green, and Spring Mint Green. Believe it or not, these organic tea bags can also be found at grocery stores.

www.stdalfour.com

ON-LINE HEALTH EDUCATION

Glyconutrients The most in depth, coherent and complete compilation of the science of glyconutrients, the essential sugars necessary for the maintenance of health.

www.glycoscience.com

Dairy – Not Milk Information regarding controversial issues surrounding milk and other dairy products.

www.notmilk.com

Institute for Health Freedom An honest source for information about policies that affect your freedom to choose your health care treatments and providers and to maintain your health privacy including genetic privacy.

www.forhealthfreedom.org

International Coalition for Drug Awareness A source for researching the dangers of many prescription drugs.

www.drugawareness.org

The Weston A. Price Foundation A wonderful source for education on nutrition, farming and the healing arts.

www.westonaprice.org

American Iatrogenic Association Medical errors are the third leading cause of death in the United States. In fact, one out of every five drug prescriptions in the typical hospital is wrong. But medical errors are the not only way that consumers are harmed. The Centers for Disease Control and Prevention estimates that 2 million people annually acquire infections while hospitalized and 90,000 people die from those infections. This is a website promoting accountability for medical professionals and institutions and reporting of illness.

www.iatrogenic.org

NUTRITION EDUCATION RESOURCE

International Foundation for Nutrition and Health The International Foundation for Nutrition and Health is a non-profit educational organization reaching out to health care professionals. IFNH collects and disseminates unique information on nutrition and whole food concentrates. It is our belief that the research on nutrition and health prior to the 1940s was done with natural whole foods, whereas the research done after World War II has been done with synthesized chemical by-products. It is also our belief that there is no reason to re-invent the wheel, the answers to all our health needs are well stated and documented in many earlier works.

3963 Mission Blvd.
San Diego, CA 92109
Phone: 1-858-488-8932
Fax: 1-858-4880-2566

www.ifnh.org

International Ministry of Health and Healing Dedicated to the freedom of health, religion and understanding that the power that made the body heals the body.

www.imhh.net

So that we may share your success stories, please send us your triumphs with
Glyco-Meridian Therapy to:

Sano Press
1930 Village Center Circle
Suite 3-177
Las Vegas, NV 89134

Or email: triumphs@sanoinstute.org

So that we may share your success stories, please send us
your triumphs with
Glyco-Meridian Therapy to:

Sano Press
1930 Village Center Circle
Suite 3-177
Las Vegas, NV 89134

Or email: triumphs@sanoinstute.org

THE SANO
INSTITUTE, Inc.

1930 Village Center Circ #3-177
Las Vegas, NV 89134
Phone 702.233.6702 Fax 702.233.6720
www.sanoclinic.com

ORDER
FORM

Ordered By (Billing Address):

Name _____

Company _____

Address _____

City, State ZIP _____

Phone _____

Ship To: (if Different than Ordered By)

Name _____

Company _____

Address _____

City, State ZIP _____

Phone _____

QTY	Item#	DESCRIPTION	UNIT PRICE	TOTAL
	ISM-49	Book "In Search of Manna" ISBN: 0-9743151-0-9 (S&H $5.00 first book; $3.00 ea. additional book).	$49.00	

SUBTOTAL	
NV res 7.5% Sales Tax	
SHIPPING & HANDLING	
OTHER	
TOTAL	

Visa ☐   MasterCard ☐

Credit
Card#   _____

Expiration
Date   _____

1. Send Check or Fax Credit Card Information
    to above address.
2. **Checks payable to Sano Institute, Inc.**
3. Web Ordering: www.marmapoint.com
4. Volume discounts call 702.233.6702

_____   _____
Authorized by   Date